AOSpine Masters Series

Metastatic Spinal Tumors

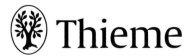

AOSpine Masters Series

Metastatic Spinal Tumors

Series Editor:
Luiz Roberto Vialle, MD, PhD
Professor of Orthopedics, School of Medicine
Catholic University of Parana State
Spine Unit
Curitiba, Brazil

Guest Editors:
Ziya L. Gokaslan, MD, FACS
Donlin M. Long Professor
Professor of Neurosurgery, Oncology, and Orthopaedic Surgery
Director, Neurosurgical Spine Program
Vice Chair, Department of Neurosurgery
Johns Hopkins University School of Medicine
Baltimore, Maryland

Charles G. Fisher, MD, MHSc, FRCSC
Professor and Head
Division of Spine Surgery
Department of Orthopaedic Surgery
University of British Columbia
Vancouver, British Columbia

Stefano Boriani, MD
Unit of Oncologic and Degenerative Spine Surgery
Rizzoli Orthopedic Institute
Bologna, Italy

Thieme
New York • Stuttgart • Delhi • Rio

Thieme Medical Publishers, Inc.
333 Seventh Ave.
New York, NY 10001

Executive Editor: Kay Conerly
Managing Editor: Judith Tomat
Editorial Assistant: Haley Paskalides
Senior Vice President, Editorial and Electronic Product Development: Cornelia Schulze
Production Editor: Barbara A. Chernow
International Production Director: Andreas Schabert
International Marketing Director: Fiona Henderson
Director of Sales, North America: Mike Roseman
International Sales Director: Louisa Turrell
Vice President, Finance and Accounts: Sarah Vanderbilt
President: Brian D. Scanlan
Compositor: Carol Pierson, Chernow Editorial Services, Inc.

Library of Congress data is available from the publisher.

Important note: Medicine is an ever-changing science undergoing continual development. Research and clinical experience are continually expanding our knowledge, in particular our knowledge of proper treatment and drug therapy. Insofar as this book mentions any dosage or application, readers may rest assured that the authors, editors, and publishers have made every effort to ensure that such references are in accordance with **the state of knowledge at the time of production of the book.**

Nevertheless, this does not involve, imply, or express any guarantee or responsibility on the part of the publishers in respect to any dosage instructions and forms of applications stated in the book. **Every user is requested to examine carefully** the manufacturers' leaflets accompanying each drug and to check, if necessary in consultation with a physician or specialist, whether the dosage schedules mentioned therein or the contraindications stated by the manufacturers differ from the statements made in the present book. Such examination is particularly important with drugs that are either rarely used or have been newly released on the market. Every dosage schedule or every form of application used is entirely at the user's own risk and responsibility. The authors and publishers request every user to report to the publishers any discrepancies or inaccuracies noticed. If errors in thiswork are found after publication, errata will be posted at www.thieme.com on the product description page.

Some of the product names, patents, and registered designs referred to in this book are in fact registered trademarks or proprietary names even though specific reference to this fact is not always made in the text. Therefore, the appearance of a name without designation as proprietary is not to be construed as a representation by the publisher that it is in the public domain.

Printed in China by Everbest Printing Ltd.
5 4 3 2 1
ISBN 978-1-62623-046-0

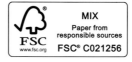

Also available as an e-book:
eISBN 978-1-62623-048-4

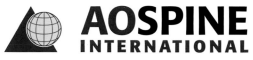

AOSpine Masters Series

Luiz Roberto Vialle, MD, PhD
Series Editor

Contents

Foreword

With the large number of publications, journals, and textbooks available to the spine practitioner, it is refreshing to see a novel publication in a new format that has a specific focus on relevant and important contemporary topics. With the introduction of the AOSpine Masters Series and the first volume focused on metastatic spinal tumors, new ground is broken on an innovative collection of educational material from the world's experts in the spine surgery field.

I congratulate all the editors and the authors of AOSpine Masters Series and the inaugural volume for their unique vision in creating this series that collects the vast knowledge of the top experts in the field. The AOSpine Masters Series addresses current topics, targeting not only our large spine surgeon membership, but also spine practitioners on a global basis. It is not a journal or a conventional book, but a publication for the world's experts to share their personal views and recommendations on a given topic. The goal of this series is to contribute to an evolving, dynamic model of an evidence-based medicine approach to spine care. Not only is the information contained in this series and in the first volume new, but the presentation of the material is truly revolutionary. The process involves a synthesis of best available evidence and consensus expert opinions to arrive at appropriate recommendations for patient care. There is no other source that combines this information or presents it in such a format for spine surgeons to approach the diseases of the spine. The foundation for treatments of the disease process is presented, with clinical pearls and complications avoidance, and an update on the current literature and key articles. I am especially excited for young spine surgeons and for residents and fellows in training programs, because this textbook will enable them to learn about spine surgery in a unique way that will provide them with a better understanding of the current status of our knowledge of the spine.

The authors are all knowledgeable experts who are world-renowned in their field. The editors who have created this vision should be congratulated and very proud of this very impressive collection of experts and the unique method of presentation. The entirety of the chapters come together to form an educational treatment focus on the individual topics. The entire collection forms an amazing series of truly master's level information that is unparalleled. I am very excited by the AOSpine Masters Series and look forward to future volumes.

Jeffrey C. Wang, MD
Chairman, AOSpine International
Chief, Orthopaedic Spine Service
Co-Director USC Spine Center
Professor of Orthopaedic Surgery and
Neurosurgery
USC Spine Center
Los Angeles, California

Series Preface

Spine care is advancing at a rapid pace. The challenge for today's spine care professional is to quickly synthesize the best available evidence and expert opinion in the management of spine pathologies. The AOSpine Masters Series provides just that—each volume in the series delivers pathology-focused expert opinion on procedures, diagnosis, clinical wisdom, and pitfalls, and highlights today's top research papers.

To bring the value of its masters level educational courses and academic congresses to a wider audience, AOSpine has assembled internationally recognized spine pathology leaders to develop volumes in this Masters Series as a vehicle for sharing their experiences and expertise and providing links to the literature. Each volume focuses on a current compelling and sometimes controversial topic in spine care.

The unique and efficient format of the Masters Series volumes quickly focuses the attention of the reader on the core information critical to understanding the topic, while encouraging the reader to look further into the recommended literature.

Through this approach, AOSpine is advancing spine care worldwide.

Luiz Roberto Vialle, MD, PhD

Guest Editors' Preface

To practice evidence-based spine surgery, a spine surgeon must combine a rigorous and critical approach to the evaluation of the scientific literature with clinical expertise and a strong commitment to patient centeredness and humanistic values. Patients with metastatic disease of the spine are a very unique patient entity for spine surgeons or any care providers; these patients are dying, and their quality of life for their remaining time is a very precious and personal process. Shared decision making in the care of these patients is essential, and often these decisions are agonizing as the physician strives to do the best, without doing "too much." From palliative or hospice care to major surgery, the goal of this book is to provide guidance for clinicians to make the right decisions and direct the best level of care possible for metastatic spine patients.

In metastatic spine disease, technologic advancements and high-quality literature on neurologic recovery, cost-effectiveness, stability, and health-related quality of life (HRQOL) have strengthened surgery's role in its management; however, choosing the correct treatment remains a challenge. Similarly on the oncology side, new radiation technologies, such as stereotactic radiosurgery have changed the treatment paradigm; formally radioresistant tumors are now radiosensitive, negating the need for high-risk surgical procedures. New, targeted molecular drugs are allowing metastatic patients to live longer, thus changing traditional decision aids for metastatic spine patients, especially for lung and renal cancer patients. Organizing and understanding all of these new concepts and technologies from a decision-making perspective is one of the major goals of this book.

The chapters have been researched and written by key opinion leaders in spine oncology and range from evaluation and decision-making principles to a spectrum of nonoperative and operative treatment options that hich have been evolving at a rapid pace, especially over the last decade. The three guest editors have reviewed each chapter to ensure consistency and the necessary synthesis of the best-available literature and expert opinion. Furthermore, a conscious and very necessary effort to ensure multidisciplinary appraisal and input has been taken. In fact, the input of the medical and radiation oncologists and radiology interventionalists, along with that of the spine surgeon, is emphasized throughout this book, just as it should be in the day-to-day care of spine metastases patients. Multiple authors were encouraged for each chapter to ensure the most balanced, transparent, and comprehensive representation possible.

Currently, there is a true paradigm shift occurring in the management of metastatic spine disease. Successful treatment must accomplish pain palliation, preservation, or recovery of neurological function and spine stability. Furthermore, with increased life expectancy, local control is gaining importance. The ultimate goal in the treatment of this fragile patient population is related to improvement in HRQOL, while limiting adverse events. We hope this guide framed around best available literature, clinical expertise, and patient preferences, will help ensure that this goal is achieved as management continues to evolve at an exciting pace.

Charles G. Fisher, MD, MHSc, FRCSC
Stefano Boriani, MD
Ziya L. Gokaslan, MD, FACS

Contributors

Mark H. Bilsky, MD
Department of Neurosurgery
Memorial Sloan-Kettering Cancer Center
New York, New York

Stefano Boriani, MD
Unit of Oncologic and Degenerative Spine
    Surgery
Rizzoli Orthopedic Institute
Bologna, Italy

Eric C. Bourekas, MD
Associate Professor, Radiology, Neurology,
    and Neurological Surgery
Chief of Neurosurgery, Department of
    Radiology
Wexner Medical Center
Ohio State University
Columbus, Ohio

Eric L. Chang, MD
Professor and Chair
Department of Radiation Oncology
Keck School of Medicine of University of
    Southern California
University of Southern California Norris
    Comprehensive Center
LAC+USC Medical Center
Keck Hospital
Los Angeles, California

Dean Chou, MD
Associate Professor
Department of Neurosurgery
Spine Center
University of California–San Francisco
San Francisco, California

Michelle J. Clarke, MD
Assistant Professor
Department of Neurosurgery
Mayo Clinic
Rochester, Minnesota

Michael S. Dirks, MD
Neurosurgery Resident
Walter Reed Army Medical Center
Washington, DC

Charles G. Fisher, MD, MHSc, FRCSC
Professor and Head
Division of Spine Surgery
Department of Orthopaedic Surgery
University of British Columbia
Vancouver, British Columbia

Daryl R. Fourney, MD, FRCSC, FACS
Assistant Professor
Division of Neurosurgery
Royal University Hospital
University of Saskatchewan
Saskatoon, Saskatchewan

Ziya L. Gokaslan, MD, FACS
Donlin M. Long Professor
Professor of Neurosurgery, Oncology,
    and Orthopaedic Surgery
Director, Neurosurgical Spine Program
Vice Chair, Department of Neurosurgery
Johns Hopkins University School
    of Medicine
Baltimore, Maryland

Ilya Laufer, MD
Department of Neurosurgery
Memorial Sloan-Kettering Cancer Center
Department of Neurological Surgery
Weill Cornell Medical College
New York, New York

Yan Michael Li, MD, PhD
Neurosurgical Fellow and Staff
M.D. Anderson Cancer Center
Houston, Texas

Ioan Adrian Lina, MD
Medical Student
University of Maryland School of
    Medicine
Department of Neurosurgery
Johns Hopkins University School
    of Medicine
Baltimore, Maryland

Simon S. Lo, MD
Associate Professor
Department of Radiation Oncology
University Hospitals Seidman
    Cancer Center
Case Comprehensive Cancer Center
Cleveland, Ohio

Ehud Mendel, MD, FACS
Tina Skestos Endowed Chair
Professor, Neurosurgery, Oncology,
    Orthopedics, and Integrated Spine
    Fellowship Program
Vice Chair, Neurosurgery Clinical Affairs
Wexner Medical Center
James Cancer Center
Ohio State University
Columbus, Ohio

Paul Porensky, MD
Neurosurgical Resident
Wexner Medical Center
Ohio State University
Department of Neurological Surgery
Columbus, Ohio

Laurence D. Rhines, MD
Professor
Department of Neurosurgery
Division of Surgery
University of Texas
M.D. Anderson Cancer Center
Houston, Texas

Arjun Sahgal, MD
Associate Professor
University of Toronto
Department of Radiation Oncology
Sunnybrook Health Sciences Centre and the
    Princess Margaret Cancer Centre
Toronto, Ontario

Rajiv Saigal, MD, PhD
Department of Neurological Surgery
University of California–San Francisco
San Francisco, California

Meic H. Schmidt, MD, MBA, FAANS, FACS
Professor of Neurosurgery and Vice Chair
    for Clinical Affairs
Ronald I. Apfelbaum Endowed Chair in
    Spine and Neurosurgery
Director, Spinal Oncology Service,
    Huntsman Cancer Institute
Director, Neurosurgery Spine
    Fellowship
Clinical Neurosciences Center
University of Utah
Salt Lake City, Utah

Daniel M. Sciubba, MD
Associate Professor of Neurosurgery,
    Oncology & Orthopaedic Surgery
Johns Hopkins University
Baltimore, Maryland

Claudio E. Tatsui, MD
Assistant Professor
Department of Neurosurgery
Division of Surgery
University of Texas
M.D. Anderson Cancer Center
Houston, Texas

Jeffrey C. Wang, MD
Chairman, AOSpine International
Chief, Orthopaedic Spine Service
Co-Director USC Spine Center
Professor of Orthopaedic Surgery and
    Neurosurgery
USC Spine Center
Los Angeles, California

Jean-Paul Wolinsky, MD
Associate Professor
Neurosurgery and Oncology
Department of Neurosurgery
Johns Hopkins University
Baltimore, Maryland

Patricia L. Zadnik, BA
Spinal Oncology Research Fellow
Sciubba Lab
Johns Hopkins Medicine
Baltimore, Maryland

1

Evaluation and Decision Making for Metastatic Spinal Tumors

Yan Michael Li, Michael S. Dirks, Claudio E. Tatsui, and Laurence D. Rhines

■ Introduction

Every year, more than 1.6 million new cases of cancer are diagnosed in the United States.[1] Roughly half of these patients eventually die from their disease, frequently due to complications from metastasis. The bone is the third most common site of metastases following lung and liver,[2] and the spine is the most common site for bone metastasis. As many as 30 to 70% of cancer patients are found to have spinal metastases on autopsy studies.[3] Symptomatic secondary metastases are estimated to occur in approximately 10 to 20% of all cancer patients.[3,4] The highest incidence of spinal metastases is found in individuals 40 to 65 years of age, corresponding to the period of highest cancer risk; 5 to 10% of patients with cancer develop spinal cord compression.[3] Up to 50% of spinal metastases require some form of treatment, and 5 to 10% require surgical management.[5] Moreover, as survival rates for many primary cancers continue to improve, it is likely that the prevalence of spinal metastases will increase.

The common tumors that spread to the spine in adults are breast, lung, prostate, renal, melanoma, thyroid, and colorectal cancers, as well as hematologic malignancies.[6–9] Multiple myeloma has the highest tendency for spinal metastases of all tumors. Spine tumors in children are represented by various forms of neuroblastoma and sarcomas.[7] There are several ways in which tumors disseminate to the spine including hematogenous spread, direct extension or invasion, and seeding of the cerebrospinal fluid. The thoracic spine is the most common site of involvement (70%), followed by the lumbar spine (20%), cervical spine, and sacrum. The vertebral body is involved in 80% of cases, with the posterior elements being affected in 20%. Most metastases are osteolytic (95%), with breast and prostate carcinomas accounting for most of the osteoblastic metastases. Occasionally both osteoblastic and osteolytic metastases occur in the same patient. Almost invariably, metastatic tumors do not involve the dura (i.e., they are epidural), but certain sarcomas and recurrent metastatic tumors after radiotherapy can violate the dural barrier.

With improvements in chemotherapy and hormonal therapy, and with the advent of novel targeted agents, medical oncologists have an increased number of therapeutic options and survival times have improved over the years. Radiotherapeutic techniques have also evolved. Spinal stereotactic radiosurgery and intensity-modulated radiation therapy (IMRT) techniques are enabling the delivery of high-dose conformal radiation to spinal tumors, erasing some of the distinction between radiosensitive and radioresistant tumor histologies. Lastly, advances in surgical techniques now enable the surgeon to treat spinal metastases more effectively than before. Spine surgery can correct mechanical instability, relieve neurologic compression, and improve pain.[9,10] Increasingly, this can be achieved through minimally invasive techniques that entail less morbidity and enable faster recovery.[11,12]

The increasing number, and complexity of, treatment modalities available for patients with spinal metastases can complicate the decision making, so the evaluation of these complex patients must be multidisciplinary, and the decision to perform surgery must be based on four key aspects of the patient's status: medical fitness, clinical presentation, oncological status, and feasibility of surgical treatment. This evaluation scheme is detailed in the remainder of this chapter. It is not meant to be an algorithm but rather a consideration of these four key aspects when developing a treatment plan for the patient with spinal metastasis and when determining the role of surgery.

■ Medical Fitness

The first fundamental consideration in managing patients with metastatic spinal disease is their overall medical condition. Many cancer patients have received prior chemotherapy or radiation, as well as steroids, and they may be malnourished from their treatment or from the disease. This may have an impact on their ability to tolerate surgical intervention.

General patient factors such as overall health, nutritional status, and medical comorbidities should all be considered in deciding whether to recommend surgery.[10] Patient factors that have been found to be related to poor surgical outcome include advanced age, obesity, malnutrition, diabetes, low bone mineral density, chronic corticosteroid use, and bone marrow suppression.[13] Hematologic status, such as leukopenia, thrombocytopenia, or coagulopathy—conditions common among cancer patients receiving chemotherapy or radiation therapy—must also be considered.

As a general rule, the more extensive the surgical procedure, the healthier the patient needs to be in order to survive the surgery and enjoy durable benefits. The patient's medical fitness may be considered not only in deciding whether to recommend surgery or not, but also in the selection of the appropriate surgical procedure and approach. Nonsurgical treatments, such as conventional radiation therapy or radiosurgery, or minimally invasive spinal procedures, such as percutaneous vertebral augmentation, may be appropriate for patients with significant medical risks or limited prognosis.

■ Clinical Presentation

The second key consideration in the management of metastatic spinal disease is the patient's clinical presentation. Patients with spinal metastases typically present with neurologic symptoms, pain, or signs of mechanical instability. It is important to recognize that the nature of the clinical presentation and the severity of the clinical findings have an impact on the choice of treatment modality.

Neurologic Function

Neurologic dysfunction is a common finding in patients with metastatic disease of the spine. A careful neurologic assessment must look for sensory and motor disturbance, autonomic dysfunction, as well as long tract signs. The main focus of the neurologic assessment is on localizing the potential lesion and determining the clinical extent of the myelopathy or the functional radiculopathy. This clinical information is then combined with the radiological evaluation to assess the degree of epidural spinal cord compression (ESCC) or nerve root compression.

Approximately 5 to 10% of patients with metastatic spine tumors develop metastatic epidural spinal cord compression (MESCC). Historically, treatment of MESCC by decompressive laminectomy alone did not provide substantial clinical benefit beyond that of conventional radiation, and it frequently further compromised spinal stability.[14,15] The development of improved surgical approaches and spinal instrumentation to treat instability has resulted in better surgical techniques for spinal decompression and stabilization.[4] Using techniques of circumferential decompression and stabilization, Patchell et al[10] conducted a randomized prospective trial of 101 patients with MESCC. They conclusively showed that early surgical decompression and stabilization followed by postoperative radiotherapy is superior to treatment with radiotherapy alone for patients with spinal cord compression caused by metastatic cancer. It should be noted that this study did not include patients with highly radiosensitive/chemosensitive tumors such as myeloma, lymphoma, and small cell lung cancer. Significantly more patients in the surgery group (84%) than in the radiotherapy group (57%) could ambulate after treatment (odds ratio [OR], 6.2; 95% confidence interval [CI], 2.0–19.8; p = 0.001). These patients were able to maintain their ambulation for a greater duration—a median of 122 days in the surgical group compared with 13 days in the radiotherapy group (p = 0.003). The need for corticosteroids and opioid analgesics was significantly reduced in the surgical group.

The degree of MESCC at the time of clinical presentation is highly variable amongst patients. The selection criteria in the Patchell study included only patients with true deformation of the spinal cord. The Spine Oncology Study Group (SOSG) has developed and validated a six-point grading system to describe the degree of ESCC based on axial T2-weighted magnetic resonance imaging (MRI) at the site of most severe compression (**Fig. 1.1**).[16] This radiological assessment can be used in combination with the neurologic examination and tumor histology to help guide treatment.

For patients with highly radiosensitive or chemosensitive tumors, nonsurgical treatment may be adequate even in cases of high-grade spinal cord compression due to the rapid response of these tumors to radiation or chemotherapy. For other solid metastatic tumors, the Patchell study suggests that high-grade (grade 2 or 3) MESCC is best treated with surgical decompression and stabilization followed by radiation therapy. For patients who do not have significant myelopathy or functional radiculopathy with low-grade MESCC (grade 1c or less), surgery may not be necessary (unless there is significant spinal instability; see below). In this case chemotherapeutic or radiotherapeutic options (including spinal radiosurgery for radioresistant histologies) can be utilized. The nature and severity of the neurologic and radiological findings clearly influence the choice of treatment.[17]

Pain

Metastatic spine tumors most commonly come to attention with the development of pain. This occurs in 83 to 95% of patients and typically precedes the development of other neurologic symptoms.[18] It is important to recognize that

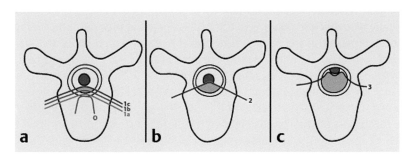

Fig. 1.1a–c Schematic representation of the 6-point epidural spinal cord compression (ESCC) grading scale[16]. Grade 0, tumor is confined to bone only. **(a)** Grade 1, tumor extension into the epidural space without deformation of the spinal cord. This is further divided into 1a, epidural impingement but no deformation of the thecal sac; 1b, deformation of the thecal sac without spinal cord abutment; and 1c, deformation of the thecal sac with spinal cord abutment but no compression. **(b)** Grade 2, spinal cord compression but cerebrospinal fluid (CSF) is visible. **(c)** Grade 3, spinal cord compression without visible CSF. Grades 0, 1a, and 1b are considered for radiation as first treatment in the lack of mechanical instability. Grades 2 and 3 define high-grade ESCC. Note: Used with permission from Bilsky MH, Laufer I, Fourney DR, et al. Reliability analysis of the epidural spinal cord compression scale. J Neurosurg Spine 2010;13(3):324–328.

there are different types of pain caused by metastatic spine tumors, and the nature of the pain may impact decision making. There are three types of pain that affect patients with symptomatic spinal metastases: local or biological, radicular, and mechanical.

Local pain is thought to result from periosteal stretching, elevation of endosteal pressure, or inflammation caused by tumor growth.[19] The pain can be localized, is often constant, and presents in the evenings and mornings. It is described as a deep "gnawing" or "aching" pain at the site of disease; it does not worsen with movement and may improve with activity. This type of pain is quite responsive to anti-inflammatory or corticosteroid medications, and radiation therapy can relieve it by shrinking the tumor and decreasing the production of inflammatory mediators.

Radicular pain is caused by nerve root impingement, which occurs when a spinal metastases compresses the exiting nerve root within the spinal canal, within the neuroforamen, or outside the foramen. The radicular pain follows a dermatomal distribution and is described as sharp, shooting, or stabbing in nature. It is often constant and may or may not be relieved with changing position. As with local pain, radicular pain may respond to therapies that can reduce the effective size of the tumor, including corticosteroids, chemotherapy, and radiation therapy.

Mechanical pain is severe and movement-related. It typically worsens with loading of the spine as a patient moves from lying down to sitting and from sitting to standing. Bending often exacerbates the pain, and it is relieved with recumbency. It is typically associated with vertebral collapse, as the weakened vertebra is no longer able to support the mechanical loads placed on it. It is important when assessing spine tumor patients to evaluate their pain when they are sitting or standing, because mechanical pain might not be noted in patients lying in bed. Mechanical pain must be distinguished from local and radicular pain. It is often refractory to anti-inflammatory medications, chemotherapy, and radiation. Although these modalities may treat the underlying tumor, they are not effective at restoring the mechanical integrity of the spine, and therefore are unlikely to provide durable relief of mechanical pain. Patients with mechanical pain typically require a treatment aimed at strengthening the affected spinal region, such as cement augmentation or spinal stabilization.

Mechanical Instability

The final component of the clinical evaluation is to recognize the patient presenting with spinal instability. The SOSG has defined neoplastic spinal instability as the "loss of spinal integrity as a result of a neoplastic process that is associated with movement-related pain, symptomatic or progressive deformity, and/or neural compromise under physiologic loads."[20] Mechanical instability due to spinal metastasis is an indication for surgical stabilization or percutaneous vertebral augmentation, regardless of the ESCC grade or the chemo/radiosensitivity of the tumor. Although effective for local tumor control, chemotherapy and radiation therapy have little or no impact on spinal stability. As a result, patients with gross neoplastic spinal instability generally require a surgical intervention.

The assessment of spinal instability is based on a combination of both clinical and radiographic information. The SOSG has proposed a set of criteria, the Spine Instability Neoplastic Score (SINS) (**Table 1.1**),[20] to help clinicians evaluate instability. This grading scheme is based on six parameters: location of the lesion, presence and type of pain, radiographic alignment, nature of the lesion (lytic or blastic), vertebral body collapse, and posterior element involvement. Each parameter receives a numerical score. Metastatic spine lesions with a low SINS (0–6) are generally considered stable and do not require surgical intervention, whereas a high SINS (13–18) suggests instability that is likely to require surgical stabilization. Intermediate SINS (7–12) tumors are considered potentially unstable and represent the middle of the instability spectrum. The SINS does not recommend any specific treatment but is a guide to help both surgeons and nonsurgeons recognize those patients who might be at risk for progressive vertebral collapse and deformity. The SINS demonstrated near perfect inter- and

Table 1.1 The Spinal Instability Neoplastic Score (SINS)

SINS Component	Description	Score
Location	Junctional (occiput-C2, C7-T2, T11-L1, L5-S1)	3
	Mobile spine (C3-C6, L2-L4)	2
	Semi-rigid (T3-T10)	1
	Rigid (S2-S5)	0
Pain[a]	Yes	3
	Occasional pain but not mechanical	1
	Pain-free lesion	0
Bone lesion	Lytic	2
	Mixed (lytic/blastic)	1
	Blastic	0
Radiographic spinal alignment	Subluxation/translation present	4
	De novo deformity (kyphosis/scoliosis)	2
	Normal alignment	0
Vertebral body collapse	> 50% collapse	3
	< 50% collapse	2
	No collapse with > 50% body involved	1
	None of the above	0
Posterolateral involvement of spinal elements[b]	Bilateral	3
	Unilateral	1
	None of the above	0

[a] Pain improvement with recumbency and/or pain with movement/loading of the spine.
[b] Facet, pedicle or costovertebral joint fracture or replacement with tumor.
Source: From Fisher CG, DiPaola CP, Ryken TC, et al. A novel classification system for spinal instability in neoplastic disease: an evidence-based approach and expert consensus from the Spine Oncology Study Group. Spine 2010;35:E1221–E1229. Reproduced with permission.

intraobserver reliability in determining the three clinically relevant categories of stability: stable (SINS 0–6), potentially unstable (SINS 7–12), and unstable (SINS 13–18). The sensitivity and specificity for detecting potentially unstable or unstable lesions were 95.7% and 79.5%.[13]

■ Oncological Status

The third key element of the evaluation of the patient with spinal metastatic disease is oncological status. Most importantly this includes recognition of the specific tumor histology. In addition, the extent of metastatic disease (bone, visceral) and the extent and nature of prior treatment also have an impact on the management of the spine metastasis.

Histology

It is critical to identify the tumor histology because it provides important information about the patient's prognosis. In fact, the histology of the primary tumor is the single strongest predictor of postoperative survival in patients undergoing surgery for spinal metastases.[21,22] According to Tomita et al,[21] tumor histologies can be stratified into three groups: slow-growing tumors, including breast, prostate, thyroid, and carcinoid tumors; moderately growing tumors, including those arising from the kidney and uterus; and rapidly growing tumors, including tumors of the lung, liver, stomach, esophagus, pancreas, bladder, sarcoma, and tumors of unknown origin. In general, the more aggressive the histology, the worse the prognosis.

Knowledge of the tumor histology also provides critical information regarding the responsiveness of the spinal metastasis to nonsurgical therapies such as chemotherapy and radiation therapy. The impact of chemotherapy and radiotherapy varies considerably with tumor type.[23,24] Chemotherapy is generally reserved for asymptomatic or minimally symptomatic lesions because its effects typically take time to manifest and this may be problematic for symptomatic patients. The obvious exceptions to this are the hematologic malignancies or Ewing's sarcoma, which may respond rapidly to chemotherapy. In patients without neurologic deficit or spinal instability, it may be perfectly reasonable to utilize systemic therapy for sensitive histologies. Breast and prostate cancers, for example, can be quite sensitive to hormonal therapies.[25,26]

With regard to radiation, tumors have traditionally been considered radiosensitive or radioresistant depending on their response to conventional radiation therapy (CRT).[23,24] Without precise conformal technique, the dosing of CRT is limited by spinal cord tolerance, as the cord is within the radiation field that is used to treat the tumor. Hence, a tumor that responds favorably to doses limited by cord tolerance is considered radiosensitive, whereas those that do not respond favorably to these doses are considered radioresistant. In cases where the tumor is in close proximity to the spinal cord, it may be impossible to radiate the tumor without radiating the cord, and the radiosensitivity of the tumor, therefore, will determine whether this modality can be used effectively. Most authors consider lymphoma, myeloma, and seminoma to be highly radiosensitive and treatable with CRT even in cases of spinal cord compression. Of the solid tumors, breast, prostate, ovarian, and neuroendocrine carcinomas are considered to be radiosensitive, whereas renal, thyroid, hepatocellular, non–small-cell lung, colon, melanoma, and sarcoma are considered radioresistant.[17] Spinal stereotactic radiosurgery (SRS), which can be used to deliver highly conformal doses of radiation to spinal tumors while avoiding the spinal cord, has been shown to provide excellent tumor control in a histology-independent manner.[13,24,27] However, this technique is limited when the tumor and spinal cord are in close proximity.

Finally, it is important to identify the tumor type, as certain histologies are particularly hypervascular. Metastases from renal cell, thyroid, hepatocellular, melanoma, and giant cell tumors can all bleed substantially during tumor resection. Preoperative embolization can be very effective in reducing intraoperative blood loss.[28] One must identify hypervascular tumors preoperatively in order to take advantage of this procedure.

To confirm the histology in a patient with a spinal tumor, percutaneous biopsy may be required. This is not generally necessary when a patient with a known primary and active metastatic disease presents with a new spinal lesion. However, when there is no known primary or when a patient with a known primary has been without active disease for a prolonged interval, biopsy should be strongly considered in order to confirm the diagnosis, to exclude a second primary, or to rule out a primary bone tumor. This may be particularly true in patients who have a history of prior chemotherapy or radiation, which may increase the chance of a second malignancy.

Extent of Metastatic Disease/ Systemic Staging

In addition to the type of tumor, the presence and extent of extraspinal metastatic disease have an impact on decision making. The presence of additional visceral and bone metastases adversely affects survival, which in turn may have an impact on the choice of treatment.[21,22] This is the basis for the well-known Tomita scoring system, which assigns point values to these three factors to generate a score, which in turn determines the aggressiveness of treatment. Grade of malignancy (slow growth, 1 point; moderate growth, 2 points; rapid growth, 4 points), visceral metastases (no metastasis, 0 points; treatable, 2 points: untreatable, 4 points), and bone metastases (solitary or isolated, 1 point; multiple, 2 points) are used to generate a score from 2 to 10. A prognostic score of 2 to 3 points indicates a wide or marginal excision for long-term local control; 4 to 5 points indicates marginal or intralesional excision for middle-term local control; 6 to 7 points indicates palliative surgery for short-term palliation; and 8 to 10 points indicates nonoperative supportive care for end of life. Cancer therapies have evolved considerably since the publication of this paper. As a result the treatments recommended based on the prognostic score may no longer be optimal. Nonetheless, the impact of these prognostic factors on survival is clear. Patients with extensive systemic disease have a poorer survival and are less likely to benefit from major surgical procedures. Moreover, the increased disease burden may cause comorbidities (e.g., decreased pulmonary function from lung metastasis, coagulopathy from liver metastasis), that render the patient less able to tolerate larger procedures. Therefore, staging is mandatory and should be performed in all patients prior to surgery, if possible.

It is worth noting the aforementioned prognostic factors characterized by Tomita; tumor histology, visceral metastasis, and bone metastasis, are also components of the well-known Tokuhashi scoring system. In their system, Tokuhashi et al[22] consider six key prognostic factors: general condition, number of extraspinal bone metastases, number of metastases in the vertebral body, presence or absence of metastases to major internal organs, site of the primary lesion, and severity of palsy. In addition to the primary site of the cancer (tumor histology), they evaluate presence of metastases to the major internal organs and score these as irremovable, removable, and none. They separate bone metastases into extraspinal and vertebral classifying the former as ≥ 3, 1 to 2, or 0, and the latter as ≥ 3, 2, or 1. Finally, they stratify the general condition of the patient (Karnovsky Performance Status) as poor (10–40), moderate (50–70), or good (80–100), and the presence of spinal cord palsy as complete, incomplete, or none. Each parameter is then assigned a range of scores to provide a maximum total of 15. The score is then used to determine how aggressive a treatment to select. Patients with lower scores are recommended for more conservative approaches, with higher scoring patients receiving excisional surgeries. The consistency rate between the criteria for predicted prognosis and the actual survival period was high in patients within each score range (0–8, 9–11, or 12–15), 86.4% in the 118 patients evaluated prospectively after 1998, and 82.5% in all 246 patients evaluated retrospectively. The prognostic criteria scoring system were useful for predicting the prognosis irrespective of treatment modality or local extension of the lesion.

Extent of Previous Treatment

The final component of the patient's oncological status is the nature and extent of the prior therapy. This is not easy to stratify or quantify, and it needs to be evaluated on a patient-by-patient basis; however, the concept is relatively self-evident. Simply put, when considering treatment options for a patient with spinal metastatic disease, the choice will be influenced by what therapies have already been utilized and the relative efficacy of the remaining treatment strategies. As an illustrative example, a patient has metastatic breast cancer and a midthoracic lesion that is abutting the cord, causing some mild radiculopathy but no neurologic dysfunction. If this patient is therapy naïve, treatment options may include conventional radiotherapy, hormonal/chemotherapy (depending on receptor status), or surgery. But if this lesion has been previously irradiated and the patient is receiving third-line chemotherapy, nonsurgical options may be limited, and surgery may be necessary if the prognosis is reasonable. The presence and proximity of prior radiation fields is often a determining factor regarding the efficacy or feasibility of subsequent radiation due to issues of spinal cord tolerance. Spinal SRS may help to minimize cord toxicity but requires that there be some degree of spatial separation between the tumor and the neurologic structures.[24,29] Clearly, patients who have received multiple prior therapies may be further along in their overall disease trajectory. This may reflect a decreased overall prognosis that must be considered prior to surgery.[17,18] Collaboration among the medical oncology, radiation oncology, and surgical teams is necessary to develop optimal treatment plans for these complicated patients.

■ Feasibility of the Surgical Plan

The final factor that must be considered before intervening surgically for a spinal metastasis is the feasibility of the surgical plan. The goal of treatment for spinal metastatic disease is palliation. Surgery must be able to reduce pain, restore and protect neurologic function, and restore spinal stability in a manner that is durable over the remaining life expectancy of the patient and with acceptable morbidity. Quality of life should be enhanced. There is ample evidence to suggest that surgery can help to achieve these goals, and in certain circumstances, particularly in the case of MESCC, may be the superior treatment option. In the case of high-grade MESCC, when combined with postoperative radiation, surgery provides far superior outcomes than does radiation alone.[9,10,30] Moreover, surgery may be the only means of correcting symptomatic spinal instability. Lastly, surgery may be the best option in cases where chemotherapeutic and radiotherapeutic strategies have failed or are otherwise limited. However, surgery also tends to be among the most invasive treatments for spinal metastases and carries significant potential for complications. This is particularly relevant in a patient population that may have substantial comorbidities related to advanced age; underlying disease; prior treatment with chemotherapy, radiation therapy, or steroids; and poor nutritional status.[7,31,32]

In short, it is the responsibility of the spinal surgeon to carefully consider the surgical plan prior to taking a patient to the operating room. First, the surgeon must consider the strategy for resection of the metastasis. Will the resection be intralesional or en bloc? Given the palliative nature of surgery for metastatic disease, most resections are performed in a piecemeal fashion. However, there are some circumstances (indolent histology, solitary spinal metastasis, long predicted survival) where a more aggressive en bloc resection may be considered.[33] In addition, for hypervascular histologies, a preoperative embolization should be considered to reduce intraoperative blood loss.[28]

Second, the surgeon must consider the surgical approach. Often this is a matter of individual preference; however, there are certainly regional anatomic constraints that may influence this decision, and these are discussed in a subsequent chapter.[13,34] There may also be factors related to the individual patient that influence the choice of surgical approach. For example, the surgeon may wish to avoid operating in a previously radiated or operated site in order to reduce wound healing complications and make the dissection easier.[31] Alternatively, it may not be feasible to consider a transthoracic approach in a patient with compromised pulmonary function. It is imperative for the surgeon to consider whether an access surgeon with additional expertise might provide a safer and more satisfactory surgical approach.

Third, the surgeon must consider the strategy for spinal reconstruction and stabilization. There are numerous devices, materials, and techniques that are available for rebuilding the spine following resection of a spinal metastasis. It is beyond the scope of this chapter to review this topic or the biomechanical principles of spinal reconstruction. However, there is one important point that the spine surgeon must contemplate in the spinal metastasis patient— the quality of the patient's bone. The stability of a spinal reconstruction and stabilization relies on the implants contacting and fixating into bone of satisfactory quality. When this is not the case, implants can loosen and fixation can be compromised, leading to spinal instability. The presence of tumor in adjacent or nearby vertebra is one factor that can impact fixation. Imaging studies should be scrutinized to make sure that there is limited tumor burden in vertebra that is being relied on to provide adequate structural support. In addition, osteopenia and osteoporosis are common among cancer patients.[35] This may be a by-product of advanced age, female sex, or treatments for the underlying cancer including steroids, chemotherapy, hormonal therapy, and radiotherapy. Poor nutritional status may also lead to bone loss. The spine surgeon must recognize this potential problem and avoid surgery, alter the reconstruction plan technique, or consider the adjunctive use of vertebral augmentation to improve the strength of the vertebra and fixation.

Lastly, the spine surgeon must consider wound healing. A palliative spine surgery that decompresses the neurologic elements and stabilizes the spine is not successful if the patient is left with a nonhealing wound. This can lead to a prolonged hospital stay and, more importantly, can delay the administration of much-needed systemic therapy. It is incumbent upon the surgeon to recognize factors that will impede healing. These include prior radiation or surgery, chemotherapy, steroids, and malnutrition. Obviously, if previous radiation and surgical fields can be avoided, this is advantageous.[31] However, this is often not the case. If the surgery is elective, there may be time to discontinue chemotherapy or steroids and improve the nutritional status of the patient. Unfortunately, most surgeries for spinal metastatic disease are done under more urgent circumstances. Therefore, the surgeon is frequently left with a situation that requires surgery, but presents wound healing challenges. In these situations, we strongly recommend collaboration with a plastic surgeon for immediate flap reconstruction at the time of the surgical resection and stabilization.[36,37] The utilization of local muscle advancement flaps, rotational flaps, and even free tissue transfer at the time of the initial spine surgery can dramatically reduce complications related to wound healing.

Consideration of these aforementioned factors when planning surgery for spinal metastatic disease will help avoid poorly conceived operations, reduce complications, and lead to improved patient outcomes.

■ Treatment Algorithms

Utilizing the principles of evaluation and decision making outlined in this chapter, several authors and institutions have developed algorithms for the management of patients with spinal metastases. Obviously, treatment decisions must be made on an individual basis and not all patients will fit neatly within any procedural framework. Moreover, each institution will base its algorithm on the treatment modalities available within that center. Nonetheless, it is instructive to see how the key factors described above are integrated into two of the most commonly utilized treatment algorithms for patients with metastatic disease to the spine. These are the Algorithm for Spinal Metastases (**Fig. 1.2**) developed and prospectively applied by Boriani's group in Bologna since January 2002,[38–40] and the neurologic, oncological, mechanical, and systemic (NOMS) decision framework (**Fig. 1.3**) utilized during the past 15 years at Memorial Sloan-Kettering Cancer Center.[17]

In both treatment paradigms, a critical initial assessment is the overall medical status of the patient. In the Boriani algorithm, this is referred to as operability, and in the NOMS it is the systemic assessment. Those patients unable to tolerate surgery are referred for radiation or medical therapy. The next critical factor is the clinical presentation. In both frameworks the degree of neurologic compromise (measured either neurologically or by the degree of spinal cord compression) directs a patient toward surgery unless the histology is highly sensitive to chemotherapy or conventional radiation. Similarly, the presence of spinal instability (risk of pathological fracture in Boriani) leads the patient toward a surgical remedy. The oncological status of the patient is tightly intertwined with the clinical presentation. In particular, the impact of the tumor histology on response to radiation and chemotherapy is a critical factor. Chemo- and radiosensitive histologies are more likely to be managed with nonsurgical modalities as long as there is no worsening neurologic compromise or spinal instability. Resistant histologies are directed toward surgery by Boriani's algorithm. In NOMS, these tumors may be treated by spinal SRS (not available in Bologna) if the degree of cord compression is low grade. For high-grade compression with radioresistant histology, separation surgery to remove the compressive portion of the tumor and stabilize the spine, followed by radiosurgery to the remaining disease, is rec-

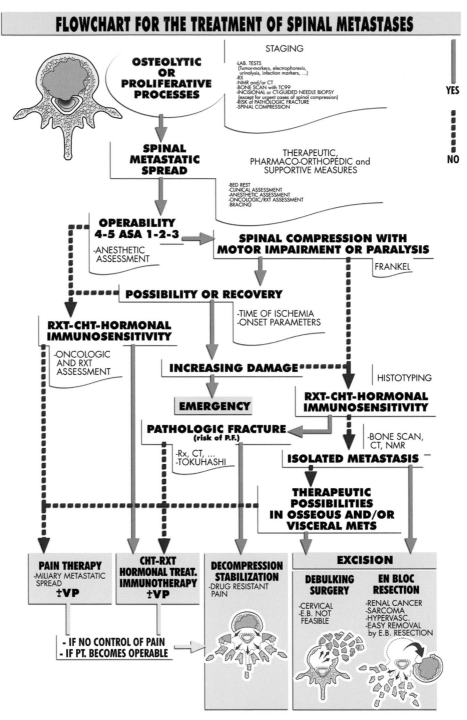

Fig. 1.2 Boriani's Treatment algorithm for spinal metastasis. ASA, American Society of Anesthesiologists; CHT, chemotherapy; CT, computed tomography; E.B., en bloc; Frankel, Frankel grading system; METS, metastases; NMR, nuclear magnetic resonance; PT., patient; RXT, radiation therapy; VP, vertbroplasty. (From Cappuccio M, Gasbarrini A, Van Urk P, Bandiera S, Boriani S. Spinal metastasis: a retrospective study validating the treatment algorithm. Eur Rev Med Pharmacol Sci 2008;12: 155–160. Reproduced with permission.)

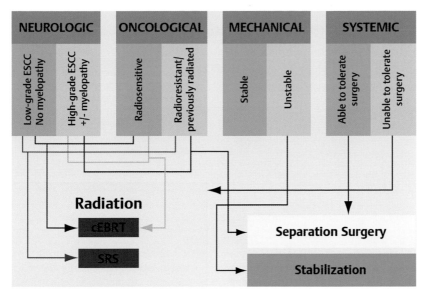

Fig. 1.3 Schematic description of the neurologic, oncological, mechanical, and systemic (NOMS) decision framework.[17,29] cEBRT, conventional external beam radiation; ESCC, epidural spinal cord compression; SRS, stereotactic radiosurgery.

(Adapted from Laufer I, Rubin DG, Lis E, et al. The NOMS framework: approach to the treatment of spinal metastatic tumors. Oncologist 2013;18: 744–751.)

ommended.[29] Implicit in both of these frameworks is that the surgeons carefully consider the feasibility of any treatment plan in advance of its execution.

■ Chapter Summary

The appropriate management of patients with metastatic spinal disease requires an appreciation for the complexity of this challenging clinical condition. Spine surgeons who treat patients with tumors not only need to be experts in the technical aspects of performing spinal surgery, but also must have an understanding of oncological principles and nonsurgical treatments available for these patients. This chapter reviewed the literature that serves as the basis for evaluation and decision making in the management of patients with metastatic spinal disease. The factors relevant to a patient's medical fitness to undergo surgery were discussed, as was evaluation of common clinical

presenting symptoms, including pain, neurologic dysfunction, and mechanical instability. This chapter also discussed evaluation of a patient's oncologic status and the feasibility of surgery as part of the treatment plan. Commonly used management algorithms were reviewed. After reading this chapter, the reader should have a basic understanding of the many factors that need to be taken into consideration when developing a plan to manage a patient with metastatic spinal disease.

Pearls

- ◆ Manage spine tumor patients as part of a multidisciplinary team.
- ◆ Understand what you are treating. Whenever possible, obtain a tissue diagnosis before operating on a spine tumor.
- ◆ Have a well-thought-out operative plan. Consider factors such as the need to stage procedures, the need for approach surgeons, and the need for plastic surgeons. Have a plan for spinal reconstruction and stabilization.

Pitfalls

- Unnecessary or excessive surgery: Understand the patient's prognosis and other treatment options available. Avoid major operations on patients with limited life expectancy or potential for recovery.
- Problems with wound healing: Consider using a plastic surgeon for local flap reconstruction. Use drains when necessary. Pay attention to nutrition in the postoperative period. Implement a mobilization strategy to avoid pressure ulcers.

- Operating without a tissue diagnosis: Tumor histology provides critical information regarding prognosis, availability of adjuvant therapies, type of surgery required, and need for embolization. Most patients who present with metastatic spine tumors do not need emergent surgery. Most will achieve significant relief of symptoms with steroids. In the vast majority of cases there is time to establish the tissue diagnosis, obtain appropriate multidisciplinary evaluation, and carefully plan surgery.

References

Five "Must-Read" References

1. Cancer Facts and Figures 2013. American Cancer Society, 2013. http://www.cancer.org/acs/groups/content/@epidemiologysurveilance/documents/document/acspc-036845.pdf.
2. Aaron AD. The management of cancer metastatic to bone. JAMA 1994;272:1206–1209
3. Jacobs WB, Perrin RG. Evaluation and treatment of spinal metastases: an overview. Neurosurg Focus 2001;11:e10
4. Sundaresan N, Digiacinto GV, Hughes JE, Cafferty M, Vallejo A. Treatment of neoplastic spinal cord compression: results of a prospective study. Neurosurgery 1991;29:645–650
5. Bilsky MH, Lis E, Raizer J, Lee H, Boland P. The diagnosis and treatment of metastatic spinal tumor. Oncologist 1999;4:459–469
6. Constans JP, de Divitiis E, Donzelli R, Spaziante R, Meder JF, Haye C. Spinal metastases with neurological manifestations. Review of 600 cases. J Neurosurg 1983;59:111–118
7. Choi D, Crockard A, Bunger C, et al; Global Spine Tumor Study Group. Review of metastatic spine tumour classification and indications for surgery: the consensus statement of the Global Spine Tumour Study Group. Eur Spine J 2010;19:215–222
8. Hatrick NC, Lucas JD, Timothy AR, Smith MA. The surgical treatment of metastatic disease of the spine. Radiother Oncol 2000;56:335–339
9. Ibrahim A, Crockard A, Antonietti P, et al. Does spinal surgery improve the quality of life for those with extradural (spinal) osseous metastases? An international multicenter prospective observational study of 223 patients. Invited submission from the Joint Section Meeting on Disorders of the Spine and Peripheral Nerves, March 2007. J Neurosurg Spine 2008;8:271–278
10. Patchell RA, Tibbs PA, Regine WF, et al. Direct decompressive surgical resection in the treatment of spinal cord compression caused by metastatic cancer: a randomised trial. Lancet 2005;366:643–648
11. Kan P, Schmidt MH. Minimally invasive thoracoscopic approach for anterior decompression and stabilization of metastatic spine disease. Neurosurg Focus 2008;25:E8
12. Gottfried ON, Dailey AT, Schmidt MH. Adjunct and minimally invasive techniques for the diagnosis and treatment of vertebral tumors. Neurosurg Clin N Am 2008;19:125–138
13. Paton GR, Frangou E, Fourney DR. Contemporary treatment strategy for spinal metastasis: the "LMNOP" system. Can J Neurol Sci 2011;38:396–403
14. Otsuka NY, Hey L, Hall JE. Postlaminectomy and post-irradiation kyphosis in children and adolescents. Clin Orthop Relat Res 1998;354:189–194
15. Fourney DR, Abi-Said D, Rhines LD, et al. Simultaneous anterior-posterior approach to the thoracic and lumbar spine for the radical resection of tumors followed by reconstruction and stabilization. J Neurosurg 2001;94(2, Suppl):232–244
16. Bilsky MH, Laufer I, Fourney DR, et al. Reliability analysis of the epidural spinal cord compression scale. J Neurosurg Spine 2010;13:324–328
17. Laufer I, Rubin DG, Lis E, et al. The NOMS framework: approach to the treatment of spinal metastatic tumors. Oncologist 2013;18:744–751
18. Sciubba DM, Petteys RJ, Dekutoski MB, et al. Diagnosis and management of metastatic spine disease. A review. J Neurosurg Spine 2010;13:94–108
19. Gokaslan ZL. Spine surgery for cancer. Curr Opin Oncol 1996;8:178–181
20. Fisher CG, DiPaola CP, Ryken TC, et al. A novel classification system for spinal instability in neoplastic disease: an evidence-based approach and expert consensus from the Spine Oncology Study Group. Spine 2010;35:E1221–E1229
21. Tomita K, Kawahara N, Kobayashi T, Yoshida A, Murakami H, Akamaru T. Surgical strategy for spinal metastases. Spine 2001;26:298–306
22. Tokuhashi Y, Matsuzaki H, Oda H, Oshima M, Ryu J. A revised scoring system for preoperative evaluation

of metastatic spine tumor prognosis. Spine 2005; 30:2186–2191

23. Maranzano E, Latini P. Effectiveness of radiation therapy without surgery in metastatic spinal cord compression: final results from a prospective trial. Int J Radiat Oncol Biol Phys 1995;32:959–967

24. Gerszten PC, Mendel E, Yamada Y. Radiotherapy and radiosurgery for metastatic spine disease: what are the options, indications, and outcomes? Spine 2009; 34(22, Suppl):S78–S92

25. Janni W, Hepp P. Adjuvant aromatase inhibitor therapy: outcomes and safety. Cancer Treat Rev 2010;36: 249–261

26. Payne H, Khan A, Chowdhury S, Davda R. Hormone therapy for radiorecurrent prostate cancer. World J Urol 2013;31:1333–1338

27. Damast S, Wright J, Bilsky M, et al. Impact of dose on local failure rates after image-guided reirradiation of recurrent paraspinal metastases. Int J Radiat Oncol Biol Phys 2011;81:819–826

28. Roscoe MW, McBroom RJ, St Louis E, Grossman H, Perrin R. Preoperative embolization in the treatment of osseous metastases from renal cell carcinoma. Clin Orthop Relat Res 1989;238:302–307

29. Laufer I, Iorgulescu JB, Chapman T, et al. Local disease control for spinal metastases following "separation surgery" and adjuvant hypofractionated or high-dose single-fraction stereotactic radiosurgery: outcome analysis in 186 patients. J Neurosurg Spine 2013;18: 207–214

30. Villavicencio AT, Oskouian RJ, Roberson C, et al. Thoracolumbar vertebral reconstruction after surgery for metastatic spinal tumors: long-term outcomes. Neurosurg Focus 2005;19:E8

31. Ghogawala Z, Mansfield FL, Borges LF. Spinal radiation before surgical decompression adversely affects outcomes of surgery for symptomatic metastatic spinal cord compression. Spine 2001;26:818–824

32. Mazel C, Balabaud L, Bennis S, Hansen S. Cervical and thoracic spine tumor management: surgical indications, techniques, and outcomes. Orthop Clin North Am 2009;40:75–92, vi–vii vi–vii.

33. Murakami H, Kawahara N, Demura S, Kato S, Yoshioka K, Tomita K. Total en bloc spondylectomy for lung cancer metastasis to the spine. J Neurosurg Spine 2010;13:414–417

34. Fourney DR, Gokaslan ZL. Use of "MAPs" for determining the optimal surgical approach to metastatic disease of the thoracolumbar spine: anterior, posterior, or combined. Invited submission from the Joint Section Meeting on Disorders of the Spine and Peripheral Nerves, March 2004. J Neurosurg Spine 2005; 2:40–49

35. Coleman RE, Lipton A, Roodman GD, et al. Metastasis and bone loss: advancing treatment and prevention. Cancer Treat Rev 2010;36:615–620

36. Vitaz TW, Oishi M, Welch WC, Gerszten PC, Disa JJ, Bilsky MH. Rotational and transpositional flaps for the treatment of spinal wound dehiscence and infections in patient populations with degenerative and oncological disease. J Neurosurg 2004;100(1, Suppl Spine):46–51

37. Garvey PB, Rhines LD, Dong W, Chang DW. Immediate soft-tissue reconstruction for complex defects of the spine following surgery for spinal neoplasms. Plast Reconstr Surg 2010;125:1460–1466

38. Gasbarrini A, Cappuccio M, Mirabile L, et al. Spinal metastases: treatment evaluation algorithm. Eur Rev Med Pharmacol Sci 2004;8:265–274

39. Cappuccio M, Gasbarrini A, Van Urk P, Bandiera S, Boriani S. Spinal metastasis: a retrospective study validating the treatment algorithm. Eur Rev Med Pharmacol Sci 2008;12:155–160

40. Gasbarrini A, Li H, Cappuccio M, et al. Efficacy evaluation of a new treatment algorithm for spinal metastases. Spine 2010;35:1466–1470

2

Neoplastic Spinal Instability

Daryl R. Fourney and Charles G. Fisher

■ Introduction

Restoration or maintenance of spinal stability is an important objective in the surgical treatment of spinal metastasis, but is often neglected in settings of neurologic compromise. Indeed, a prospective randomized trial has demonstrated the superiority of surgery and radiation therapy compared to radiation therapy alone in the management of high-grade spinal cord compression for solid tumors.[1] Spinal instability is a common and distinct indication for surgery or vertebral augmentation with vertebroplasty or kyphoplasty.[2] However, it has not been studied as rigorously as spinal cord compression. This reflects the controversy that exists regarding tumor-related instability. The biomechanical and clinical literature in this area is remarkably limited.[3] Prior to the Spinal Instability Neoplastic Score, there were few clinical criteria published, and none had been tested for reliability or validity. The lack of standardized criteria led to significant variation with regard to diagnosis and treatment indications. In essence if the problem was not clearly defined, it was very difficult to study. The concept of spinal instability, however, remains a critical and essential component in the surgical decision-making process.

Most often, spine surgeons rely on clinical experience to determine if instability is present. Although challenging for the spine surgeon, the diagnosis of instability is even more difficult for the nonsurgeon (radiologist, oncologist), potentially leading to inappropriate referrals or patients with instability being under treated, risking pain, deformity, or neurologic deterioration.

This chapter reviews some of the principles of biomechanics as they relate to patterns of instability and deformity that occur in neoplastic disease, describes and applies the SINS in illustrative cases, and discusses the unique anatomic and biomechanical features of the different regions of the spine and options for management.

■ Principles

Definition of Tumor-Related Spine Instability

Unlike the appendicular skeleton, the spine presents a very complex environment in which to judge tumor-related instability. Metastatic cancer alters both the material and geometric properties of the bone—the two entities that form the structural property rigidity. Although these properties determine the resistance to axial bending and twisting loads in bone, the "bone" or vertebra's resistance to load in the spine is unique and significantly influenced by the region and adjacent anatomy. Indeed, there can be fracture or collapse in the spine, but no clinical symptoms, deformity, or fracture progression. The infinite complexity has led to a simpler approach in trying to define and predict spinal in stability in the setting of metastatic disease. The Spine Oncology Study Group (SOSG) defines spine instability as loss of spinal integrity as a result of a neoplastic process that is associated with movement-related pain, symptomatic or progressive deformity, or neural compromise under physiological loads.[4]

Basic Biomechanical Principles in Spine Tumors Versus Trauma

Tumor-related instability is very distinct from high-energy traumatic injuries in the pattern of bony and ligamentous involvement, neurologic manifestations, and bone quality. In addition, the ability of the spine to heal is compromised by the tumor, systemic therapies, irradiation, and the general biological compromise of these patients.[5]

Principle 1: Load Sharing

Disease that involves the cancellous core of the vertebral body with preservation of the cortical bony support may not result in instability. Taneichi et al[6] analyzed radiological and clinical data from patients with thoracic and lumbar metastases and created a multivariate logistic regression model to identify the probability of collapse under various states of tumor involvement. They found that in the thoracic spine, destruction of the costovertebral joint was a more important risk factor for collapse than the size of the metastatic lesion within the vertebral body, presumably related to loss of stiffness and strength normally provided by the rib cage. In the thoracolumbar and lumbar spine, the most important factor for collapse was the size of the vertebral body defect. Involvement of the pedicle had a much greater influence on vertebral collapse compared with the thoracic spine. Other studies have suggested that bone mineral density is more important than defect size in predicting fracture threshold.

Principle 2: Tension Band

Anterior compressive forces are balanced by a posterior system composed of muscles and ligaments working under tension. The well-vascularized vertebral bodies are the most common sites of tumor involvement, with posterior vertebral elements being much less frequently affected. In general, the dorsal ligamentous complex is less commonly disrupted by neoplasm as compared with high-velocity trauma.[5] Iatrogenic destruction of posterior elements by laminectomy is probably more common than disruption by the tumor itself. Destruction of the facet joints by tumor is also rarer than in trauma, but when it is present, it may result in significant translational or rotational deformity.

Impending Collapse

The biomechanical effects of spinal metastases are poorly defined. As a result, there are no standards for predicting the risk of pathological fracture, even when lesions have been identified and characterized with modern imaging studies. Theoretically, vertebral body collapse may be prevented by radiation therapy or systemic therapies if the tumor is sensitive to one of those treatments and its growth (and therefore lytic destruction of the vertebra) can be arrested. Once the tumor reaches a critical size, which may be defined as "impending collapse," only surgical prophylactic stabilization (e.g., percutaneous cement, pedicle screws) can prevent fracture. Unfortunately, a reliable method to predict impending collapse does not exist due to the regional biomechanical and anatomic issues. Therefore, treatment of instability should generally be on the basis of actual clinical instability rather than asymptomatic or relatively asymptomatic radiological findings that imply the potential for instability in the future.

Spinal Instability Neoplastic Score

In the SINS classification system, tumor-related instability is assessed by adding together six individual component scores: spine location, pain, lesion bone quality, radiographic alignment, vertebral body collapse, and posterolateral involvement of the spinal elements (see **Table 1.1**). Each component of SINS has demonstrated clinically acceptable reliability.[7]

The minimum score is 0 and the maximum is 18. Total SINS scores have near-perfect inter- and intraobserver reliability when collapsed into three clinically relevant assessments of tumor-related instability, which can be described as stability (0–6), indeterminate instability (potentially unstable) (7–12), and instability (13–18). Surgical consultation is recommended for patients with SINS scores ≥ 7. Examples of scoring are presented in **Figs. 2.1, 2.2**, and **2.3**.

Content and face validity of the SINS was facilitated by integrating the best evidence provided by two systematic reviews with expert consensus from members of the SOSG.[4] At the time of this writing, there are no prospective studies that have assessed SINS. However, a retrospective validity analysis found that the false-negative rate was low (4.3%), and all of these type II errors were due to distinguishing stable from potentially unstable cases (not stable vs unstable).[7]

When Is Vertebroplasty or Kyphoplasty Sufficient for Stabilization?

Assigning a numerical grade to instability (SINS 0–18) is attractive because it recognizes that, unlike in trauma, spinal stability due to tumor is not lost suddenly in an "all-or-none" fashion. Instead, it is gradual process that at a certain point results in pathological fracture. By being able to reliably define the severity of instability we may come closer to understanding the indications for less invasive forms of stabilization such as vertebroplasty or kyphoplasty. We propose that patients with intermediate grades of instability (SINS 7–12) are more likely to be appropriate candidates for percutaneous cement, whereas those with higher scores may be better treated with spinal instrumentation.[8] Vertebral augmentation is particularly useful in patients with limited life expectancy, patients who are too medically frail to have open surgery, and patients with very poor bone quality (e.g., myeloma bone disease).[9]

Treatment of Instability by Spinal Region

Craniovertebral Junction

Metastasis in this region rarely cause myelopathy because the upper cervical canal is large, and because tumors in this region typically present with severe mechanical neck pain before they become large enough to significantly compress the spinal cord. Therefore, ventral tumor resection (via a transoral or extraoral approach) is rarely indicated, and our surgical management strategy has focused on posterior spinal stabilization.[10] We favor occipitocervical fixation over short-segment approaches because it protects the patient against the potential loss of stability due to progression of the destructive process. Our goal is to obtain a durable construct so that the use of any cumbersome and poorly tolerated external orthoses (e.g., rigid collar or halo vest) can be avoided.

Subaxial Cervical Spine

From C3 through C6, corpectomy reconstructed with a cage and plate is the most common approach. A combined anterior/posterior stabilization is often necessary for multilevel disease, circumferential tumor involvement, severe instability/deformity, and poor bone quality. Supplemental posterior stabilization is often required at the C7/T1 junction.[11]

Thoracic and Lumbar Spine

Anterior approaches are not feasible in most patients from T2 to T5, due to the great vessels and the heart. Posterolateral approaches (costotransversectomy or lateral extracavitary approach) are recommended for this region, and are also increasingly popular from T6 through L5 (as compared with anterior approaches), because they allow removal of the tumor and the application of spinal instrumentation as a single-stage operation.[12] Regardless of the approach used, the vertebral body may be reconstructed with various materials, including allograft bone, polymethylmethacrylate (PMMA), or metal cages. The latter include distractible

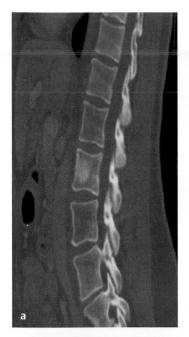
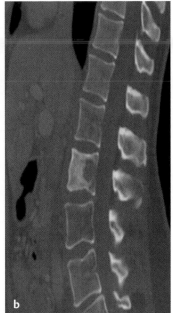
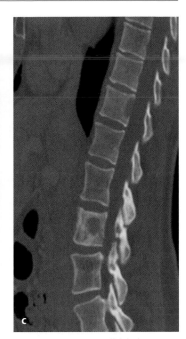
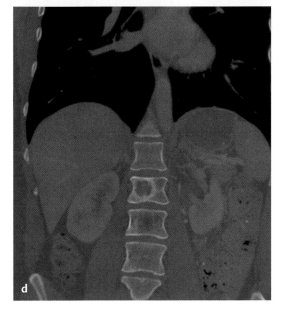
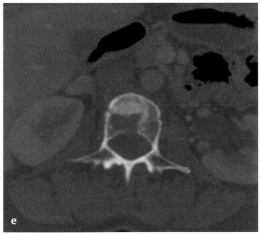

Fig. 2.1a–e Computed tomography (CT) images of **(a)** select left parasagittal view, **(b)** select midline sagittal view, **(c)** select right parasagittal view, **(d)** representative coronal view, and **(e)** axial view at L2 of a 42-year-old woman with known metastatic breast cancer who had an asymptomatic L2 lesion identified as an incidental finding on CT imaging. She denies any back pain. The Spine Instability Neoplastic Score (SINS) is calculated as follows: mobile spine location (L2), 2 points; pain-free lesion, 0 points; mixed lytic/blastic lesion, 1 point; normal spinal alignment, 0 points; no vertebral body collapse but > 50% body involvement, 1 point; no posterolateral spinal element involvement, 0 points. Total SINS = 2 + 0 + 1 + 0 + 1 + 0 = 4 (stable lesion).

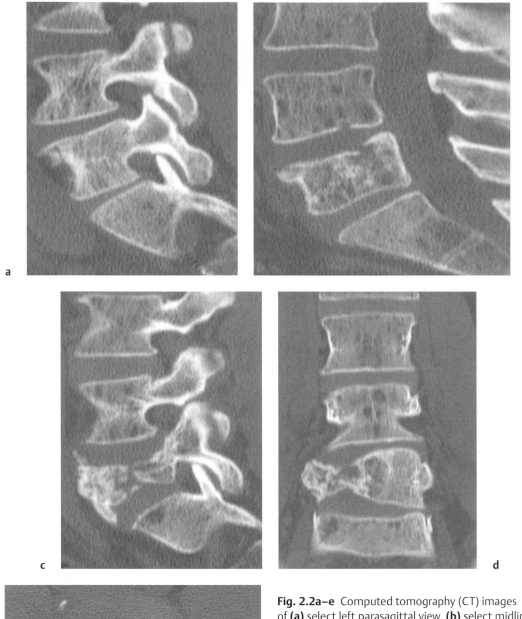

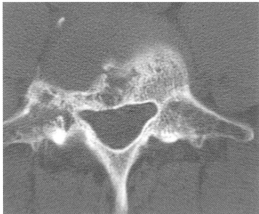

Fig. 2.2a–e Computed tomography (CT) images of **(a)** select left parasagittal view, **(b)** select midline sagittal view, **(c)** select right parasagittal view, **(d)** representative coronal view, and **(e)** axial view of a L5 lesion in a 49-year-old man with multiple myeloma who presents with mild low back pain that is not aggravated by activities or movement. The SINS is calculated as follows: junctional location, 3 points; pain but not mechanical, 1 point; lytic, 2 points; spinal alignment preserved, 0 points; < 50% vertebral body collapse, 2 points; unilateral replacement of right pedicle with tumor, 1 point. Total SINS = 3 + 1 + 2 + 0 + 2 + 1 = 9 (potential instability, surgical referral recommended).

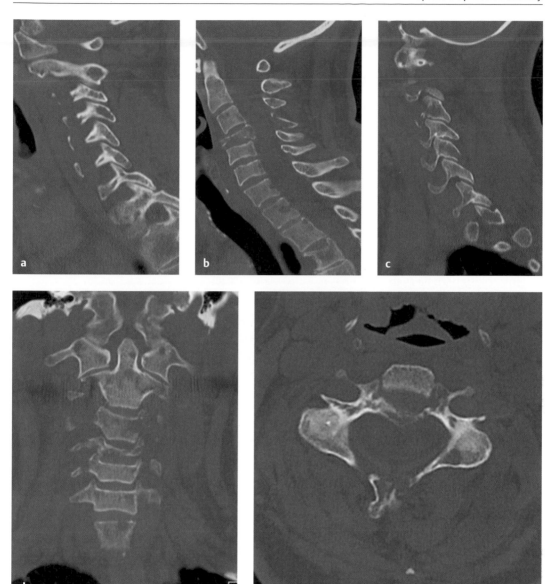

Fig. 2.3a–e Computed tomography (CT) images of **(a)** select left parasagittal view, **(b)** select midline sagittal view, **(c)** select right parasagittal view, **(d)** representative coronal view, and **(e)** axial view of a C4 lesion in a 54-year-old woman with known metastatic sarcoma who presents with neck pain exacerbated by any movement and improved with application of a cervical collar. The SINS is calculated as follows: mobile spine location, 2 points; mechanical pain, 3 points; lytic lesion, 2 points; kyphotic deformity, 2 points; > 50% collapse, 3 points; bilateral posterolateral involvement, 3 points. Total SINS = 2 + 3 + 2 + 2 + 3 + 3 = 15 (instability, surgical referral recommended).

or telescoping varieties. Polymethylmethacrylate is biologically compatible and very stable in compression, but usually requires anchoring with Steinmann pins or a chest tube. If vertebrectomy has been performed via an anterior

approach, anterior column reconstruction and stabilization with a plate without supplementary posterior stabilization may be sufficient, except in certain circumstances: significant kyphosis or deformity, such as translation; thoracolumbar junction zone; significant adjacent chest wall resection (e.g., Pancoast tumor or locally invasive sarcoma); vertebrectomy spanning two or more levels; vertebrectomy caudal to L4 (anterior fixation devices are difficult to apply in this region); and poor bone quality.[13]

Lumbosacral Junction and Sacrum

Tumors in this region, in our experience, seldom cause spondylolisthesis or other obvious deformity because the strong ligamentous support structures and the L5-S1 facet complex, which confer most of the stability in this region, are seldom completely disrupted by tumor. Although significant deformity is unusual, clinical instability with mechanical pain is not uncommon, as this region experiences the largest loads encountered in the entire spine. As with the cervicothoracic and thoracolumbar regions, the lumbosacral junction is a "high-stress" region. Relatively abrupt changes in anatomy and regional mechanics between the mobile lumbar and fixed sacral segments increase the risk of fracture and instability and present challenging problems in terms of spinal stabilization. Although sacral instability is uncommon,[14] when it is present the construct demand is high and we generally recommend providing more stability than less. We recommend large-diameter pedicle screws at S1 (7 to 8 mm), supplemented with additional sacral alar screws or iliac screws, favoring the later. With significant involvement of the sacrum and sacroiliac (SI) joints, percutaneous iliosacral or transsacral screws should be used. These can often be supplemented with cement through a small open incision.

Correction of Spinal Deformity

In general, spinal deformities that arise as a result of metastasis are secondary to collapse of the vertebral body. Therefore, with the exception of the upper cervical spine, where translational and rotational deformities may occur, neoplastic deformity is usually a kyphotic deformity. With significant chest wall disruption, or the loss of posterolateral elements (costo-vertebral joint, facet, pedicle), kyphoscoliosis may be seen. Occasionally, shearing forces may lead to spondylolisthesis.

A second feature of neoplastic deformities is that they are usually flexible. The majority may be corrected by careful positioning of the patient on the operating room table. After vertebrectomy, a distractible cage is a simple tool to correct most kyphotic deformities. Another option under the right conditions is to "shorten" the spine by compressing on normal bone once the tumor is removed—analogous to a pedicle subtraction osteotomy. Exceptions are certain upper cervical deformities (e.g., pathological dens fracture with translation, rotatory atlantoaxial subluxation), which may require the application of cervical traction.

Is Bone Fusion Necessary?

Bony fusion per se is unlikely to be achieved in many cancer patients, due to (1) limited life expectancy, (2) adjuvant chemotherapy or radiation therapy that further compromises the chance of successful fusion, or (3) poor general fitness (bone quality, nutrition, or general frailty). Our goal is to provide an immediately stable construct that minimizes or eliminates axial pain and helps to prevent neurologic deterioration during the remaining life span. In line with these principles, bracing is generally avoided as well. Allograft is often applied after stabilization in order to promote fusion for the occasional long-term survivor. However, we do not favor the use of autograft because of the potential for graft-site morbidity and the occurrence of unrecognized metastatic disease within the iliac crest bone of some patients.

■ Potential Problems

Mechanical Pain

Even in the absence of obvious vertebral body collapse or deformity, some clinical instability is assumed to be present when the syndrome of mechanical pain is present. This type of pain is characteristically aggravated by movements and improved or relieved at rest. It is important to distinguish this from local (biological) pain, which does not characteristically change with movement. Often biological pain and mechanical pain occur together in metastatic disease.

Vertebral Compression Fractures After Radiosurgery

Radiation therapy has developed new treatment paradigms over the last decade. In patients with minimal epidural disease, stereotactic body radiation therapy (SBRT) can be used to deliver radiation more precisely to the tumor, significantly reducing the dose to the spinal cord, and allowing greater dose-delivery per fraction. This advance allows durable tumor control rates independent of tumor histology-specific radiosensitivity to conventional external beam radiation therapy (cEBRT). In other words, historically "radioresistant" tumors such as renal cell carcinoma may be treated with SBRT. As well, SBRT may be used in patients in whom cEBRT has failed.

Higher doses produce superior local control but may be associated with late toxicities not associated with cEBRT, including vertebral compression fracture (VCF). Radiation myelopathy is still a rare toxicity unlike the reported data for VCF after SBRT. A series from the Memorial Sloan-Kettering Cancer Center first reported a fracture progression rate of 39% of 71 sites treated.[15] The M.D. Anderson Cancer Center later reported a rate of 20% of 123 sites treated.[16] Conversely, the risk of fracture after conventional cEBRT is only 2.8% with fractionated short-course radiation therapy (ranging most commonly from approximately 20 Gy in five fractions to approximately 30 Gy in 10 fractions).[17] Cunha et al[18] recently reported that patients treated with SBRT of 20 Gy or greater in a single fraction are at a higher risk of VCF. Vertebral augmentation with or without pedicle screw supplementation has been advocated to prevent fracture, but it is unclear which patients should receive prophylactic stabilization.

■ Chapter Summary

Many of the criteria used to define spinal stability after trauma may not be valid in the setting of oncology. Patients who develop spinal instability have, or are at high risk of having, a neurologic deficit, severe pain, and progressive deformity. An understanding of the mechanical integrity of the spine is a key component of treatment decision making in patients with metastatic disease, along with tumor histology, neurologic status, prognosis, and medical fitness for surgery. Prior to the development of the SINS, there were no accepted evidence-based guidelines for the classification of neoplastic spine instability. The SINS is the only grading system for neoplastic stability in the spine that has been shown to be reliable and valid. It is hoped that it can be used to study outcomes in an effort to clarify indications for surgical and nonsurgical treatment, especially for the intermediate grades of instability, where there is currently significant variation in practice. Because the SINS can be reliably rated by nonsurgeons (e.g., radiologists, radiation oncologists), it is hoped that it will facilitate appropriate referral patterns for surgical assessment and thus prevent unnecessary suffering and catastrophic collapse and neurologic injury.

Pearls

♦ Understand the definition of tumor-related instability and basic biomechanical principles in spine tumors.
♦ Consider "impending collapse."
♦ Utilize the Spine Instability Neoplastic Score (SINS).
♦ Appreciate when vertebral augmentation alone is sufficient for stabilization.
♦ Be aware of approaches and instrumentation for treatment of instability in each spine region.

Pitfalls

♦ Not recognizing that mechanical pain alone may be the only sign of clinical instability.
♦ High rate of vertebral compression fractures after radiosurgery.

References
Five "Must-Read" References

1. Patchell RA, Tibbs PA, Regine WF, et al. Direct decompressive surgical resection in the treatment of spinal cord compression caused by metastatic cancer: a randomised trial. Lancet 2005;366:643–648

2. Berenson J, Pflugmacher R, Jarzem P, et al; Cancer Patient Fracture Evaluation (CAFE) Investigators. Balloon kyphoplasty versus non-surgical fracture management for treatment of painful vertebral body compression fractures in patients with cancer: a multicentre, randomised controlled trial. Lancet Oncol 2011;12:225–235

3. Weber MH, Burch S, Buckley J, et al. Instability and impending instability of the thoracolumbar spine in patients with spinal metastases: a systematic review. Int J Oncol 2011;38:5–12

4. Fisher CG, DiPaola CP, Ryken TC, et al. A novel classification system for spinal instability in neoplastic disease: an evidence-based approach and expert consensus from the Spine Oncology Study Group. Spine 2010;35:E1221–E1229

5. Fourney DR, Gokaslan ZL. Spinal instability and deformity due to neoplastic conditions. Neurosurg Focus 2003;14:e8

6. Taneichi H, Kaneda K, Takeda N, Abumi K, Satoh S. Risk factors and probability of vertebral body collapse in metastases of the thoracic and lumbar spine. Spine 1997;22:239–245

7. Fourney DR, Frangou EM, Ryken TC, et al. Spinal instability neoplastic score: an analysis of reliability and validity from the spine oncology study group. J Clin Oncol 2011;29:3072–3077

8. Paton GR, Frangou E, Fourney DR. Contemporary treatment strategy for spinal metastasis: the "LMNOP" system. Can J Neurol Sci 2011;38:396–403

9. Fourney DR, Schomer DF, Nader R, et al. Percutaneous vertebroplasty and kyphoplasty for painful vertebral body fractures in cancer patients. J Neurosurg 2003;98(1, Suppl):21–30

10. Fourney DR, York JE, Cohen ZR, Suki D, Rhines LD, Gokaslan ZL. Management of atlantoaxial metastases with posterior occipitocervical stabilization. J Neurosurg 2003;98(2, Suppl):165–170

11. Fehlings MG, David KS, Vialle L, Vialle E, Setzer M, Vrionis FD. Decision making in the surgical treatment of cervical spine metastases. Spine 2009;34(22, Suppl):S108–S117

12. Polly DW Jr, Chou D, Sembrano JN, Ledonio CG, Tomita K. An analysis of decision making and treatment in thoracolumbar metastases. Spine 2009; 34(22, Suppl):S118–S127

13. Fourney DR, Gokaslan ZL. Use of "MAPs" for determining the optimal surgical approach to metastatic disease of the thoracolumbar spine: anterior, posterior, or combined. Invited submission from the Joint Section Meeting on Disorders of the Spine and Peripheral Nerves, March 2004. J Neurosurg Spine 2005;2:40–49

14. Nader R, Rhines LD, Mendel E. Metastatic sacral tumors. Neurosurg Clin N Am 2004;15:453–457

15. Rose PS, Laufer I, Boland PJ, et al. Risk of fracture after single fraction image-guided intensity-modulated radiation therapy to spinal metastases. J Clin Oncol 2009;27:5075–5079

16. Boehling NS, Grosshans DR, Allen PK, et al. Vertebral compression fracture risk after stereotactic body radiotherapy for spinal metastases. J Neurosurg Spine 2012;16:379–386

17. Chow E, Harris K, Fan G, Tsao M, Sze WM. Palliative radiotherapy trials for bone metastases: a systematic review. J Clin Oncol 2007;25:1423–1436

18. Cunha MV, Al-Omair A, Atenafu EG, et al. Vertebral compression fracture (VCF) after spine stereotactic body radiation therapy (SBRT): analysis of predictive factors. Int J Radiat Oncol Biol Phys 2012;84:e343–e349

3

Major Complications Associated with Stereotactic Ablative Radiotherapy for Spinal Metastasis

Simon S. Lo, Arjun Sahgal, and Eric L. Chang

■ Introduction

During the past decade stereotactic ablative radiotherapy (SABR), which is also known as stereotactic body radiotherapy (SBRT), has evolved as a high-dose targeted treatment aimed at local tumor control for various tumor sites such as the lung, the liver, and, now, the spine.[1] With respect to spinal metastases, it was initially developed for the re-treatment indication, as further conventional radiation was limited by the cumulative tolerance of the spinal cord, and spine SABR enables carving of the radiation dose around and away from the spinal cord to maintain safe dose limits while dose escalating the vertebral tumor segment. This technique has become a primary therapy for selected patients in the upfront setting and as postoperative therapy, and it is rapidly emerging as a commonly practiced alternative to low-dose conventional radiotherapy.[2,3] Multiple series have shown promising results with regard to local control and pain control[3]; however, as yet there are no randomized controlled trials completed to confirm superior outcomes. Radiation Therapy Oncology Group (RTOG) 0631 is an ongoing trial comparing 8 Gy in one fraction delivered conventionally to 16 to 18 Gy in one fraction delivered with SABR.

One of the major issues with this technique is the toxicity profile, which has not been extensively studied with phase 1 trials, and, moreover, there are limited prospective phase 2 trials. The fear is not so much acute toxicity but rather long-term toxicity, such as radiation myelopathy arising from overdosing the spinal cord, which is a delayed event and a devastating one for the patient, leading to paralysis, incontinence, and potentially death. This chapter summarizes the literature on adverse events with spine SABR, as several reviews have focused on clinical outcomes.[2–4]

■ Major Adverse Events

Radiation Myelopathy

Radiation myelopathy (RM) has been observed after spinal SABR in both unirradiated and re-irradiated patients. The work by Sahgal et al[5–7] at the University of Toronto has resulted in safe dose limits for both clinical situations based on the multi-institutional pooling of cases of RM and controls with no RM. For patients with no history of radiation, Sahgal et al[7] recently reported on nine cases of RM after spinal SABR and provided an unprecedented detailed dose-volume histogram (DVH) analysis. The DVH data were compared for the nine RM patients and 66 controls, and the spinal cords were contoured based on the thecal sac as a surrogate for the true cord. This contouring approach was done to factor in potential sources of error in assuming that the dose to the contoured true cord is in reality the dose that is delivered.

Sources of error include physiological spinal cord motion, intrafraction patient motion, variation in spinal cord delineation, potential errors in magnetic resonance imaging (MRI) and computed tomography (CT) image fusion, the treatment planning calculation algorithm, the image-guidance system, treatment couch motions, gantry rotation precision, and micro-multileaf collimator (mMLC) leaf position calibration. Basing the dose limits on the thecal sac essentially provides a margin of safety on the true cord that was anatomic as opposed to a fixed expansion. The authors acknowledge that this approach is roughly equivalent to a 1.5-mm margin expansion beyond the cord. All patients received SABR over one to five fractions, with fraction sizes ≥ 5 Gy. Although one patient with RM had been treated with boost SABR 6 weeks after external beam radiotherapy, the cumulative biologically effective dose (BED) was calculated. The median follow-up times for patients with and without RM was 23 and 15 months, respectively, and the median time to RM was 12 months (range, 3–15 months). In this study, all doses were converted to an equivalent BED in 2-Gy fractions, which was termed the normalized 2-Gy equivalent BED (nBED), and the α/β used for the spinal cord was 2 (hence, the dose unit is $Gy_{2/2}$). This is also known as the equivalent dose in 2 Gy fractions (EQD2). Ultimately, a model was created to yield 1%, 2%, 3%, 4%, and 5% probabilities of RM based on linear regression analysis. The doses are listed in **Table 3.1**. The authors also reported a detailed analysis of the effect of dose

within thecal sac volumes ranging from a point maximum (Pmax) to 2 cc. The most significant result was observed for the Pmax volume, corroborating the notion that the spinal cord is a serial organ.

With respect to reirradiation, Sahgal et al[6] also reported a case-control analysis based on five cases of RM and 16 controls. Once again, the thecal sac was used as a surrogate for the spinal cord. The cumulative nBED, which was defined as the sum of the nBED from the first course of conventional radiotherapy and the Pmax nBED from the SABR retreatment course for each patient was then calculated (using an α/β of 2 for the spinal cord). Based on the analysis, the authors recommended that the cumulative nBED to the thecal sac Pmax should not exceed 70 $Gy_{2/2}$, which was most applicable when the initial conventional radiotherapy nBED ranged from 30 to 50 $Gy_{2/2}$, and that the thecal sac (surrogate of spinal cord) Pmax nBED from reirradiation with SABR should not exceed 25 $Gy_{2/2}$. In addition, the model suggested that the thecal sac SABR Pmax nBED/cumulative Pmax nBED ratio should not exceed 0.5, and the minimum time interval between the two treatment courses be at least 5 months. Based on the data of this study, Sahgal et al have made recommendations on absolute dose limit for the thecal sac for re-treatment of spinal tumors with SABR (**Table 3.2**). Their colleagues at the University of Toronto follow these recommendations strictly in their high-volume centers and have not observed RM in their patients (unpublished information provided by Arjun Sahgal).

Table 3.1 Predicted Pmax Volume Absolute Doses in Gy for 1 to 5 SABR Fractions that Result in 1% to 5% Probability of Radiation Myelopathy

	1 Fraction Pmax Limit (Gy)	2 Fractions Pmax Limit (Gy)	3 Fractions Pmax Limit (Gy)	4 Fractions Pmax Limit (Gy)	5 Fractions Pmax Limit (Gy)
1% probability	9.2	12.5	14.8	16.7	18.2
2% probability	10.7	14.6	17.4	19.6	21.5
3% probability	11.5	15.7	18.8	21.2	23.1
4% probability	12.0	16.4	19.6	22.2	24.4
5% probability	12.4	17.0	20.3	23.0	25.3

Abbreviation: Pmax, maximum point dose.
Source: From Sahgal A, Weinberg V, Ma L, et al. Probabilities of radiation myelopathy specific to stereotactic body radiation therapy to guide safe practice. Int J Radiat Oncol Biol Phys 2013;85:341–347. Reproduced with permission from Elsevier.

Table 3.2 Reasonable Reirradiation SABR Doses to the Thecal Sac Pmax Following Common Initial Conventional Radiotherapy Regimens*

Conventional Radiotherapy (nBED)	1 Fraction: SABR Dose to Thecal Sac P_{max}	2 Fractions: SABR Dose to Thecal Sac P_{max}	3 Fractions: SABR Dose to Thecal Sac P_{max}	4 Fractions: SABR Dose to Thecal Sac P_{max}	5 Fractions: SABR Dose to Thecal Sac P_{max}
0	10 Gy	14.5 Gy	17.5 Gy	20 Gy	22 Gy
20 Gy in 5 fractions (30 $Gy_{2/2}$)	9 Gy	12.2 Gy	14.5 Gy	16.2 Gy	18 Gy
30 Gy in 10 fractions (37.5 $Gy_{2/2}$)	9 Gy	12.2 Gy	14.5 Gy	16.2 Gy	18 Gy
37.5 Gy in 15 fractions (42 $Gy_{2/2}$)	9 Gy	12.2 Gy	14.5 Gy	16.2 Gy	18 Gy
40 Gy in 20 fractions (40 $Gy_{2/2}$)	N/A	12.2 Gy	14.5 Gy	16.2 Gy	18 Gy
45 Gy in 25 fractions (43 $Gy_{2/2}$)	N/A	12.2 Gy	14.5 Gy	16.2 Gy	18 Gy
50 Gy in 25 fractions (50 $Gy_{2/2}$)	N/A	11 Gy	12.5 Gy	14 Gy	15.5 Gy

Abbreviations: N/A, not applicable; nBED, normalized biologically effective doses; SABR, stereotactic ablative radiotherapy.
*These dose limits are based on a prior publication by Sahgal et al. for spinal cord tolerance in patients treated with SABR and no prior history of radiation.
Source: From Sahgal A, Ma L, Weinberg V, et al. Reirradiation human spinal cord tolerance for stereotactic body radiotherapy. Int J Radiat Oncol Biol Phys 2012;82:107–116. Reproduced with permission from Elsevier.

Controversy

The recommendations of Sahgal et al were based on BED modeling to convert the various dose-fractionation schemes into a single number, as it represents at this time the easiest model to apply in the clinic with the least number of assumptions. However, the linear-quadratic (LQ) model has recently been challenged in its ability to accurately estimate the BED in the ablative dose range (> 15 Gy/fraction) as used in SABR. Wang et al[8] have proposed a generalized LQ (gLQ) model, which provides a natural extension across the entire dose range. This model was independently validated for tumor response in in-vitro studies at Thomas Jefferson University, but it had not been employed to model toxicities in normal tissues[9] until Huang et al[10] reanalyzed the data from the above discussed paper on spinal cord tolerance for reirradiation with SABR by Sahgal et al, using the gLQ model. It was also determined that no RM was observed when the cumulative Pmax nBED to the thecal sac was ≤ 70 $Gy_{2/2}$ based on conversions using the gLQ model.[10] However, with the scarcity of clinical data, the gLQ model must be approached with extreme caution, and clinical validation is necessary.

Vertebral Compression Fracture

Vertebrae bearing metastases are prone to pathological fractures due to the replacement of healthy bone with tumor. Lytic disease is inherently weaker than sclerotic disease; however, both increase the risk of skeleton-related events. Radiotherapy, frequently used as a treatment for bone metastasis, can increase the risk of fracture, but the risk is thought to be low with conventional palliative doses. However, SABR is based on ablative doses of radiation and delivered to the clinical target volume (CTV), which typically includes the entire vertebral body; hence, tumor and normal bone tissue are exposed. It is only recently that vertebral compression fracture (VCF) after spinal SABR has been reported in the literature in detail.[11–13]

Researchers at Memorial Sloan-Kettering Cancer Center (MSKCC) first reported their observation of VCF following SABR for spinal metastases. The dose regimen used was 18 to 24 Gy in one fraction, with a majority of patients receiving 24 Gy in one fraction. They observed progressive VCF in 39% of the vertebrae treated at a median time of 25 months.[13] The location of spinal metastasis (above T10 vs T10 or below), the nature of the spinal metastasis (lytic vs sclerotic and mixed), and the percentage of vertebral body involvement were identified as predictors of VCF.

Compared to the study from MSKCC, researchers at M.D. Anderson Cancer Center (MDACC)[11] and the University of Toronto[12] reported much lower rates of VCF and at an earlier time-course post-SABR (median time ranging from 2 to 3.3 months). In the MDACC study, the incidence of new or progressive VCF in 93 patients with 123 spinal metastases treated with SABR was 20%. Unlike the MSKCC study where a single-fraction regimen was used for SABR for all patients, approximately two thirds of the patients in the MDACC cohort received either 27 Gy in three fractions or 20 to 30 Gy in five fractions. Factors predicting development of VCF included age > 55 years, a preexisting fracture, and baseline pain. Obesity was found to have a protective effect. The median time to fracture progression was 3 months after SBRT. Similarly, the study from the University of Toronto, which included 90 patients with 167 spinal metastases treated with SABR, also included patients treated with two to five fractions in addition to those treated with a single fraction. The identified risk factors for VCF included the presence of kyphosis/scoliosis, lytic appearance, primary lung and hepatocellular carcinoma, and a dose per fraction ≥ 20 Gy. The crude rate of VCF was 11% and the 1-year fracture-free probability was 87.3%. The median time to fracture after SBRT was 2 months.

The much higher rate of VCF observed in the MSKCC study was likely related to the very aggressive regimen of 24 Gy in one fraction used for the majority of the patients in that study.[13] This corroborated with the finding from the University of Toronto study that a dose per fraction of ≥ 20 Gy was associated with an increased risk of VCF,[12] which implies that the radiation has an independent effect on the risk of VCF. Moreover, a clinicopathological study from the University of Toronto found that radiation necrosis of the bone is likely the under-lying mechanism of the fracture, which again makes radiobiological sense.[14] However, there was a discrepancy of the time frame within which VCF occurred between the MSKCC study and the MDACC and University of Toronto studies. The much later median time to VCF reported by the MSKCC group at 25 months versus 3 and 2 months by the MDACC and University of Toronto[11-13] may imply that with further follow-up the risk of VCF may continue to rise or that the pathological processes may be different.

Pain Flare

Pain flare, defined as a transient increase in pain during or shortly after radiotherapy, has been observed after conventional radiotherapy for bone metastasis. So far, there has been only one study addressing pain flare specific to spine SABR. Chiang et al[15] at the University of Toronto performed a prospective study examining the incidence of pain flare and the predictive factors of the complication. A total of 41 steroid-naïve patients were enrolled, and pain was assessed using the Brief Pain Inventory (BPI) at baseline, during SABR, and for 10 days after SABR. The investigators recorded the use of pain medications with dosages converted to an oral morphine equivalent dose (OMED), and the use of steroids, daily during the study period.

Pain flare was defined as

1. a 2-point increase of worst pain score on BPI with no change in oral morphine equivalent dose;
2. a 25% increase in oral morphine equivalent dose with no decrease in worst pain score; or
3. any initiation of steroid therapy.

In terms of SABR dose, 18 patients received 20 to 24 Gy in a single fraction and 23 patients received 24 to 35 Gy in two to five fractions to their spinal metastases. Pain flare was observed in 28 (68.3%) of 41 patients, with eight (28.6%) of 28 patients experiencing pain flare the day after SABR completion. Fifteen (53.6%) of 28 patients had a 2-point increase in worst pain score with no change in analgesic intake, five (17.9%) needed a 25% increase in analgesic intake with no decrease in worst pain score, and eight (28.6%) needed initiation of dexamethasone. With respect to risk factors associated with pain flare, none of the dosimetric or tumor-specific factors were predictive of pain flare. Only the Karnofsky Performance Scale (KPS) and the location of the index vertebra (cervical and lumbar) were predictive. Rescue dexamethasone at 4 mg orally once daily for the remainder of the course of SABR, or for 5 days after SABR either during or within 10 days from completion of SABR, was found to effectively treat the pain flare.

Esophageal Toxicity

The esophagus is located immediately in front of the spinal column, especially for the thoracic segments, and is susceptible to injury by ablative doses of radiation delivered to the spine. There is limited literature specific to esophageal toxicity from SABR. In a large study from MSKCC in which 182 patients with 204 spinal metastases abutting the esophagus were treated with single-fraction SBRT to a dose of 24 Gy, esophageal toxicity was scored according to the National Cancer Institute Common Toxicity Criteria for Adverse Events version 4.0.[16] There were 31 (15%) acute and 24 (12%) late esophageal toxicities during the median follow-up interval of 12 months. Grade 3 or higher acute or late toxicities were observed in 14 (6.8%) patients. For grade 3 or higher esophageal toxicities, the median splits for $D_{2.5cm3}$ (the minimum dose to the 2.5 cm^3 receiving the highest dose), V_{12} (the volume receiving at least 12 Gy), V_{15}, V_{20}, and V_{22} were 14 Gy, 3.78 cc, 1.87 cc, 0.11 cc, and 0 cc, respectively. They also note the maximum point dose should be kept below 22 Gy. Importantly, the seven patients who developed grade 4 or higher toxicities either had radiation recall reactions after chemotherapy with doxorubicin or gemcitabine, or iatrogenic esophageal manipulation, such as biopsy, dilatation, and stent placement.

In a study from Stanford University, 31 patients treated with SABR for lung or spinal tumors < 1 cm from the esophagus were reviewed to determine esophageal tolerance.[17] Treatment regimens included 16 to 25 Gy in one fraction, 8 to 12 Gy × 2 fractions, 8 Gy × 3 fractions, 6 to 12.5 Gy × 4 fractions, and 5 to 10 Gy × 5 fractions. Three of 31 patients developed esophageal toxicities and two of them died of either a tracheoesophageal fistula or esophageal perforation (grade 5). Dosimetric parameters examined included D_{5cc}, D_{2cc}, D_{1cc}, and D_{max}. When the LQ model was used to convert the dose to a single fraction, the D_{5cc}, D_{2cc}, D_{1cc}, and D_{max} for the three patients ranged from 10.7 to 16.5 Gy, 13.7 to 18.2 Gy, 15.7 to 19 Gy, and 18.5 to 22.8 Gy, respectively. When the universal survival curve (USC) model was used to convert the dose to single fraction, the corresponding numbers were 11.9 to 16.5 Gy, 17.4 to 18.2 Gy, 19 to 22.5 Gy, and 21 to 37.3 Gy, respectively. Further data and modeling are required before hard dose limits are known, but both these studies suggest keeping the maximum dose ≤ 20 Gy.

Radiation Plexopathy/ Radiculopathy

Given the close proximity of the spinal nerves and nerve plexuses to the vertebrae, these structures are susceptible to injury by ablative doses of radiation delivered through SABR. Although rare, radiation radiculopathy or plexopathy has been observed. In a phase I/II trial of single-dose SABR for radiation naïve spinal metastases from MDACC, where doses of 16 to 24 Gy were given, of 61 patients treated, 10 developed mild (grade 1 or 2) numbness and tingling and one developed grade 3 radiculopathy at L5.[18] Researchers at Beth Israel Deaconess Hospital (Boston, MA) observed four cases of persistent or new radiculopathy in their cohort of 60 patients with recurrent epidural spinal metastases treated with SABR. All of those patients had radiological progression of disease, and it is unclear whether the complications were caused by tumor progression, radiation injury of the spinal nerves, or a combination of both.[19] Investigators from MDACC observed two cases of grade 3 lumbar plexopathy in their study on reirradiation with SBRT for recurrent spinal metastases in 59 patients.[20]

The tolerance of the brachial plexus to SABR has been investigated in a study from Indiana

University, where 36 patients with 37 apical primary lung cancers were treated with a dose of 30 to 72 Gy in three or four fractions.[21] Seven cases of grade 2 to 4 brachial plexopathy was observed. The cutoff dose was determined to be 26 Gy in three or four fractions, which is in keeping with the constraint of 24 Gy in three fractions used in the RTOG trials. The 2-year rates of brachial plexopathy were 46% and 8% when the maximum brachial plexus dose was > 26 Gy and ≤ 26 Gy, respectively. One caveat of the study is that the subclavian/axillary vessels, which served as a surrogate for brachial plexus, instead of the full brachial plexus were contoured.

Avoiding Complications

To minimize the risks of serious complications caused by spinal SABR, all relevant organs at risk (OARs) such as the spinal cord, cauda equina, nerve plexuses and roots, and esophagus should be contoured and the dose constraint for each OAR should be respected. For critical neural structures such as the spinal cord and cauda equina, MRI is required for very accurate contouring.[22] Fusion of the spinal MRI (axial T1 and T2 sequences) with the treatment planning CT should be performed to facilitate the process. The quality of the fusion should be carefully checked before the image sets are used for delineation of the neural structures. In patients who cannot undergo a spinal MRI or in the postoperative setting where there is significant metallic artifacts on MRI obscuring the visualization of the spinal cord, a CT myelogram can be used for delineation of the spinal cord. It is crucial that the window leveling is correct because inaccurate window leveling will lead to inaccurate cord contouring, which in turn will result in inaccurate determination of cord dose.

Universal to SABR for all body sites and particularly for spinal tumors, robust immobilization is of the utmost importance. Most OARs including critical neural structures like the spinal cord and nerve roots are in very close proximity to the spinal CTVs, and the dose gradient between the spinal cord and spinal CTV is typically very steep in SABR for spinal metastases such that even slight deviations in positioning

may result in overdosing of those structures, leading to catastrophic neurologic complications.[5] When a linear-accelerator (LINAC)-based system is used for SABR, the use of the BodyFIX (Elekta, Stockholm, Sweden) near-rigid body immobilization system has been demonstrated by researchers at the University of Toronto to be more robust in minimizing intrafraction motions as compared to a simple vacuum cushion system, limiting the set-up error to 2 mm.[23]

Intrafraction patient motion occurs despite the application of advanced technology to its fullest extent, especially when the treatment time is anticipated to be long. Investigators from University of Toronto evaluated their LINAC-based system and showed that there could be intrafraction motion of 1.2 mm and 1 degree with near-rigid body immobilization (BodyFIX), image-guidance with kilovoltage cone-beam CT (CBCT), and a robotic couch capable of adjusting shifts with 6 degrees of freedom.[24] To maintain this level of precision, it was concluded that intrafraction repeat cone-beam CT is necessary to check for any positional variation and at an interval of approximately every 20 minutes. Newer technologies like volumetric modulated arc therapy (VMAT) and the high dose rate flattening filter-free feature can drastically reduce treatment time and may render intrafraction cone-beam CT unnecessary. With the use of a CyberKnife unit, which is capable of real-time intrafraction imaging with in-room stereoscopic kV x-ray and providing feedback to a mini-LINAC mounted on a robotic arm, a positioning accuracy of 1.0 mm and 1.0 degree can be achieved.[25] Near-rigid body immobilization may not be necessary for this system as the CyberKnife is unique in its ability to reposition the LINAC while treatment is being delivered with tight tolerances. Apart from intrafraction patient motion, physiological spinal cord motion can also contribute to uncertainties or errors in the estimation of true spinal cord dose from SABR.[5] Taking into account all the abovementioned factors, it is prudent to create a Planning organ-at-risk volume (PRV) for the spinal cord to decrease the risk of RM caused by potential errors that can lead to overdosing of the spinal cord. Although some institutions and RTOG do not use a PRV to set a dose constraint for spinal cord, the authors routinely use the thecal sac or a 1.5- to 2.0-mm margin around the MRI/myelogram delineated cord to set the dose constraint for spinal cord.

Sahgal et al[6,7] have made recommendations on spinal cord dose constraints using the thecal sac as a surrogate in a radiation-naïve situation and a reirradiation setting (**Tables 3.1** and **3.2**). As mentioned above, one of the authors (Sahgal), who follows these recommendations strictly, has not observed any incident of RM, having treated at least 500 targets over the last 5 years. Alternatively, spinal cord dose constraints of 10 Gy in five fractions and 9 Gy in three fractions have been used by the other two authors (Lo and Chang) in the reirradiation setting, with prior conventional radiotherapy dose ≤ 45 Gy (1.8–2.0 Gy per fraction), and RM has not been observed. The reanalysis of the data on spinal cord tolerance for reirradiation with SABR using the gLQ model has yielded interesting results, which are different from those of the original study.[10] However, extensive clinical validation is necessary to guide safe treatment. Currently, the data from the original study by Sahgal et al. represent the best clinical data available.[6]

As mentioned above, several risks factors have been identified, predicting VCF after SABR for spinal metastases. It seems to be prudent to avoid using a single fraction of ≥ 20 Gy,[12] especially for patients with the above-mentioned risk factors. In patients with preexisting fractures, prophylactic kyphoplasty or vertebroplasty before SABR can be offered and may reduce the risk of further fracture and palliate the mechanical pain to enable the patient to tolerable subsequent SABR. For pain flare, rescue steroids are effective, and the use of prophylactic steroids may be best, subject to a further study at the University of Toronto. Medrol Pak Oral (Pfizer, Brooklyn, NY) is a commercially available prepacked version of methylprednisolone that is more convenient for patients to use during SABR.

The esophagus is immediately anterior to the vertebral column mostly in the lower cervical and thoracic regions, and it is expected that some portions of the esophagus will receive a proportion of the dose delivered to the spinal metastasis. Therefore, it is crucial to contour the esophagus as an OAR and to respect its tolerance in order to minimize the risk of serious complications. Data from MSKCC showed that the maximum dose tolerated was volume-dependent, as mentioned above.[16] Other factors that increase the risk of severe esophageal toxicity such as post-SABR doxorubicin- or gemcitabine-based chemotherapy or surgical esophageal manipulation should be avoided if possible. The use of a multiple session regimen (three to five fractions) may also decrease the risk of esophageal injury by SABR if the dose constraint cannot be met in one fraction.

Nerve plexuses and nerve roots are susceptible to injury by ablative radiation.[18-20] To spare these structures, they need to be carefully and accurately contoured. These structures can be better visualized on MRI, which can be fused with treatment planning CT. Best efforts must be made to respect the dose constraints of these neural structures, especially at levels where the nerves roots or nerve plexuses are responsible for motor function of the extremities. The contouring atlas of brachial plexus is available at the RTOG website (http://www.rtog.org/CoreLab/ContouringAtlases/BrachialPlexusContouringAtlas.aspx).

Table 3.3 lists the constraints used by RTOG trials for the spinal cord, esophagus, cauda equina, and nerve plexuses. Note that the constraints in the table have not been tested clinically, and their use outside of a clinical trial setting is not authorized by RTOG.

■ Chapter Summary

The major complications that have been observed after SABR for spinal metastases include RM, VCF, pain flare, esophageal toxicity, and nerve injury.[6,7,11-20] Given the proximity of those relevant OARs to the vertebrae, these complications are not unexpected. Every effort must be made to spare those structures from doses beyond their tolerance. Robust near-rigid immobilization and strategies to manage intrafraction patient motion are crucial steps in safe delivery of SABR. Apart from near-rigid immo-

Table 3.3 Normal Tissue Constraints used by RTOG trials (www.rtog.org) *

Organ at Risk	1 Fraction	3 Fractions	4 Fractions	5 Fractions
Spinal cord	RTOG 0631 and 0915: 14 Gy (< 0.03 cc or maximum)/10 Gy (< 0.35 cc)/ 7 Gy (< 1.2 cc) (only for RTOG 0915)	RTOG 0236 and 0618: 18 Gy (maximum) RTOG 1021: 21.9 Gy (maximum)/ 18 Gy (< 0.35 cc)/12.3 Gy (< 1.2 cc)	RTOG 0915: 26 (maximum)/ 20.8 (< 0.35 cc)/13.6 (< 1.2 cc)	RTOG 0813: 30 Gy (maximum)/ 22.5 Gy (< 0.25 cc)/13.5 Gy (< 0.5 cc)
Brachial plexus	RTOG 0631 and 0915: 17.5 Gy (< 0.03 cc or maximum)/ 14 Gy (< 3 cc)	RTOG 0236 and 0618: 24 Gy (maximum) RTOG 1021: 24 Gy (maximum)/ 20.4 Gy (< 3 cc)	RTOG 0915: 27.2 Gy (maximum)/ 23.6 Gy (< 3 cc)	RTOG 0813: 32 Gy (maximum)/ 30 Gy (< 3 cc)
Cauda equina	RTOG 0631: 16 Gy (< 0.03 cc)/ 14 Gy (< 5 cc)	Not available	Not available	Not available
Sacral plexus	RTOG 0631: 18 Gy (< 0.03 cc)/ 14.4 Gy (< 5 cc)	Not available	Not available	Not available
Esophagus	RTOG 0631: 16 Gy (< 0.03 cc)/ 11.9 Gy (< 5 cc) RTOG 0915: 15.4 Gy (maximum)/ 11.9 Gy (< 5 cc)	RTOG 0236 and 0618: 27 Gy (maximum) RTOG 1021: 25.2 Gy (maximum)/ 17.7 Gy (< 5 cc)	RTOG 0915: 30 Gy (maximum)/ 18.8 Gy (< 5 cc)	RTOG 0813: 105% of PTV prescription (maximum)/ 27.5 Gy (< 5 cc)

*These dose constraints have not been thoroughly tested clinically, and the authors do not assume responsibility for the use of these dose limits.

bilization, intrafraction CBCT and the use of newer technologies such as VMAT and the high dose rate flattening filter-free mode to drastically reduce treatment time can also tackle intrafraction patient motion.

To facilitate accurate contouring of the spinal cord, a spinal MRI or a CT myelogram should be fused with the treatment planning CT.[22] Because of various sources of potential error, including inherent technical uncertainties and physiological spinal cord motion, there is a risk of overdosing of the spinal cord given the steep dose gradient from the spinal CTV. Although many institutions and RTOG use only the spinal cord contours to set dose constraints, it is prudent to create a safety margin for the spinal cord during treatment planning. Common practices include an expansion of a 1.5- to 2.0-cm margin around the cord contour to generate a

PRV for planning or simply the utilization of the thecal sac contours as a surrogate for the spinal cord.[3,5,22] The current recommendations for spinal cord constraints were derived based on the use of thecal sac as a surrogate.

Vertebral compression fracture occurs more commonly in patients with certain risk factors.[11–13] The most important treatment factor is the dose per fraction; the prescribed dose is ≥ 20 Gy/fraction,[12] which in essence is the dose used for a single fraction regimen. Therefore, it is recommended that one should avoid using a single dose of ≥ 20 Gy for SABR for spinal metastasis, especially in patients with risk factors for VCF. Pain flare is a common acute complication of spinal SABR and it can be prevented with the use of a short course of prophylactic dexamethasone or methylprednisolone.[15] Severe esophageal toxicities have been observed in patients who have undergone doxorubicin- or gemcitabine-based chemotherapy or surgical esophageal manipulation after single fraction SABR.[16] One should avoid those treatments or procedures after SABR, if possible. If doxorubicin- or gemcitabine-based chemotherapy is necessary as part of the treatment plan, it is recommended that it should be given before spinal SABR. The use of a multisession SABR regimen may also decrease the risk of esophageal injury. Nerve plexuses and nerve roots are susceptible to injury by ablative radiation as delivered in spinal SABR.[18–20] To spare these structures, they need to be carefully and accurately contoured. A contouring atlas is available at the RTOG website (http://www.rtog.org/CoreLab/ContouringAtlases/BrachialPlexusContouringAtlas.aspx).

The Radiation Therapy Oncology Group has a set of dose constraints for OARs for their SABR trials (www.rtog.org), but they are largely unvalidated. More clinical data are needed before they can be adopted in routine practice.

Pearls

- All relevant organs at risk (OARs) such as the spinal cord, cauda equina, nerve plexuses and roots, and esophagus should be contoured and the dose constraint for each OAR should be respected.
- Fusion of the spinal MRI (axial T1 and T2 sequences) with the treatment planning CT should be performed to facilitate the process.
- In patients who cannot undergo a spinal MRI or in the postoperative setting where there is significant metallic artifacts on MRI obscuring the visualization of the spinal cord, a CT myelogram can be used for delineation of the spinal cord.
- The quality of the fusion should be carefully checked before the image sets are used for delineation of the neural structures.
- It is crucial that the window leveling of CT myelogram be correct.
- Robust immobilization is crucial for safe delivery of SABR for spinal metastasis, and this is best achieved with the use of a device that has a double vacuum system.
- Intrafraction positional variation can be minimized by the use of intrafraction repeat cone-beam CT and the reduction of treatment time by using VMAT and the high dose rate flattening filter-free feature.
- A CyberKnife unit is capable of real time intrafraction imaging with in-room stereoscopic kV X-ray

and providing feedback to a mini-LINAC mounted on a robotic arm, and a positioning accuracy of 1.0 mm and 1.0 degree can be achieved.
- To account for physiological cord motion, a PRV for the spinal cord is created to decrease the risk of RM caused by potential errors that can lead to overdosing of the spinal cord.
- The published data and guidelines on spinal cord constraints based on real patients may be used to guide treatment planning.[6,7,10]
- Alternatively, spinal cord dose constraints of 10 Gy in five fractions and 9 Gy in three fractions have been used by two of the authors (Lo and Chang) in the reirradiation setting, with prior conventional radiotherapy dose ≤ 45 Gy (1.8–2.0 Gy per fraction), and RM has not been observed.
- It is prudent to avoid using a single fraction of ≥ 20 Gy for SABR for spinal metastasis, especially for patients with risk factors for VCF.
- For pain flare, rescue steroids are effective and the use of prophylactic steroids may be considered.
- It is crucial to contour the esophagus as an OAR and to respect its tolerance in order to minimize the risk of serious complications from spinal SABR.
- Post-SABR doxorubicin- or gemcitabine-based chemotherapy or surgical esophageal manipulation should be avoided if possible.
- The use of a multiple session regimen (three to five fractions) may also decrease the risk of esophageal injury by SABR if the dose constraint cannot be met in one fraction.
- To spare the nerve plexuses and nerve roots, they need to be carefully and accurately contoured, preferably on MRI fused with treatment planning CT.
- Best efforts must be made to respect the dose constraints of the nerve plexuses and nerve roots, especially at levels where the nerves roots or nerve plexuses are responsible for motor function of the extremities.
- The dose constraints used in SABR trials of RTOG are largely unvalidated and should be approached with extreme caution.

Pitfalls

- If OARs such as the spinal cord, cauda equina, nerve plexuses and roots, and esophagus are not contoured during treatment planning for spinal SABR, inadvertent injury to those structures may occur, leading to serious complications if dose constraints of those OARs are exceeded.
- Accurate delineation of the spinal cord and cauda equina, which is crucial to safe delivery of spinal SABR, can be difficult without fusion of appropriate scans such as MRI of the spine with the treatment planning CT.

- ◆ Metallic artifacts can interfere with delineation of spinal cord on MRI.
- ◆ Poor-quality image fusion and improper windowing can lead to inaccurate cord contouring, which in turn will result in inaccurate determination of cord dose.
- ◆ Intrafraction patient motion and physiological spinal cord motion can lead to significant uncertainty in the actual radiation dose delivered in the spinal cord.
- ◆ There are significant uncertainties regarding the spinal cord constraints for spinal SABR in a radiation-naïve and a reirradiation setting, and these pose challenges to spinal SABR practitioners.
- ◆ Vertebral compression fracture and pain flare, both very undesirable complications, can occur with SABR for spinal metastasis.
- ◆ The esophagus is immediately anterior to the vertebral column mostly in the lower cervical and thoracic regions and is susceptible to toxicity from ablative doses of radiation delivered by SABR.
- ◆ Nerve plexuses and nerve roots are susceptible to injury by ablative radiation delivered by SABR given their proximity to the vertebrae.

References

Five Must-Read References

1. Sahgal A, Roberge D, Schellenberg D, et al; The Canadian Association of Radiation Oncology-Stereotactic Body Radiotherapy Task Force. The Canadian Association of Radiation Oncology scope of practice guidelines for lung, liver and spine stereotactic body radiotherapy. Clin Oncol (R Coll Radiol) 2012;24: 629–639
2. Sahgal A, Bilsky M, Chang EL, et al. Stereotactic body radiotherapy for spinal metastases: current status, with a focus on its application in the postoperative patient. J Neurosurg Spine 2011;14:151–166
3. Sahgal A, Larson DA, Chang EL. Stereotactic body radiosurgery for spinal metastases: a critical review. Int J Radiat Oncol Biol Phys 2008;71:652–665
4. Masucci GL, Yu E, Ma L, et al. Stereotactic body radiotherapy is an effective treatment in reirradiating spinal metastases: current status and practical considerations for safe practice. Expert Rev Anticancer Ther 2011;11:1923–1933
5. Sahgal A, Ma L, Gibbs I, et al. Spinal cord tolerance for stereotactic body radiotherapy. Int J Radiat Oncol Biol Phys 2010;77:548–553
6. Sahgal A, Ma L, Weinberg V, et al. Reirradiation human spinal cord tolerance for stereotactic body radiotherapy. Int J Radiat Oncol Biol Phys 2012; 82:107–116
7. Sahgal A, Weinberg V, Ma L, et al. Probabilities of radiation myelopathy specific to stereotactic body radiation therapy to guide safe practice. Int J Radiat Oncol Biol Phys 2013;85:341–347
8. Wang JZ, Huang Z, Lo SS, Yuh WT, Mayr NA. A generalized linear-quadratic model for radiosurgery, stereotactic body radiation therapy, and high-dose rate brachytherapy. Sci Transl Med 2010;2:39ra48
9. Ohri N, Dicker AP, Lawrence YR. Can drugs enhance hypofractionated radiotherapy? A novel method of modeling radiosensitization using in vitro data. Int J Radiat Oncol Biol Phys 2012;83:385–393
10. Huang Z, Mayr NA, Yuh WT, Wang JZ, Lo SS. Reirradiation with stereotactic body radiotherapy: analysis of human spinal cord tolerance using the generalized linear-quadratic model. Future Oncol 2013;9:879–887
11. Boehling NS, Grosshans DR, Allen PK, et al. Vertebral compression fracture risk after stereotactic body radiotherapy for spinal metastases. J Neurosurg Spine 2012;16:379–386
12. Cunha MV, Al-Omair A, Atenafu EG, et al. Vertebral compression fracture (VCF) after spine stereotactic body radiation therapy (SBRT): analysis of predictive factors. Int J Radiat Oncol Biol Phys 2012;84:e343–e349
13. Rose PS, Laufer I, Boland PJ, et al. Risk of fracture after single fraction image-guided intensity-modulated radiation therapy to spinal metastases. J Clin Oncol 2009;27:5075–5079
14. Al-Omair A, Smith R, Kiehl TR, et al. Radiation-induced vertebral compression fracture following spine stereotactic radiosurgery: clinicopathological correlation. J Neurosurg Spine 2013;18:430–435
15. Chiang A, Zeng L, Zhang L, et al. Pain flare is a common adverse event in steroid-naïve patients after spine stereotactic body radiation therapy: a prospective clinical trial. Int J Radiat Oncol Biol Phys 2013; 86:638–642
16. Cox BW, Jackson A, Hunt M, Bilsky M, Yamada Y. Esophageal toxicity from high-dose, single-fraction paraspinal stereotactic radiosurgery. Int J Radiat Oncol Biol Phys 2012;83:e661–e667
17. Abelson JA, Murphy JD, Loo BW Jr, et al. Esophageal tolerance to high-dose stereotactic ablative radiotherapy. Dis Esophagus 2012;25:623–629

18. Garg AK, Shiu AS, Yang J, et al. Phase 1/2 trial of single-session stereotactic body radiotherapy for previously unirradiated spinal metastases. Cancer 2012; 118:5069–5077

19. Mahadevan A, Floyd S, Wong E, Jeyapalan S, Groff M, Kasper E. Stereotactic body radiotherapy reirradiation for recurrent epidural spinal metastases. Int J Radiat Oncol Biol Phys 2011;81:1500–1505

20. Garg AK, Wang XS, Shiu AS, et al. Prospective evaluation of spinal reirradiation by using stereotactic body radiation therapy: The University of Texas MD Anderson Cancer Center experience. Cancer 2011;117: 3509–3516

21. Forquer JA, Fakiris AJ, Timmerman RD, et al. Brachial plexopathy from stereotactic body radiotherapy in early-stage NSCLC: dose-limiting toxicity in apical tumor sites. Radiother Oncol 2009;93:408–413

22. Lo SS, Sahgal A, Wang JZ, et al. Stereotactic body radiation therapy for spinal metastases. Discov Med 2010;9:289–296

23. Li W, Sahgal A, Foote M, Millar BA, Jaffray DA, Letourneau D. Impact of immobilization on intrafraction motion for spine stereotactic body radiotherapy using cone beam computed tomography. Int J Radiat Oncol Biol Phys 2012;84:520–526

24. Hyde D, Lochray F, Korol R, et al. Spine stereotactic body radiotherapy utilizing cone-beam CT image-guidance with a robotic couch: intrafraction motion analysis accounting for all six degrees of freedom. Int J Radiat Oncol Biol Phys 2012;82:e555–e562

25. Ma L, Sahgal A, Hossain S, et al. Nonrandom intrafraction target motions and general strategy for correction of spine stereotactic body radiotherapy. Int J Radiat Oncol Biol Phys 2009;75:1261–1265

4

En Bloc Resection in the Treatment of Spinal Metastases: Technique and Indications

Ilya Laufer, Jean-Paul Wolinsky, and Mark H. Bilsky

■ Introduction

The principles of primary musculoskeletal tumor excision were thoroughly detailed by William Enneking et al.[1] Although treatment concepts applicable to primary and metastatic tumors differ, the Enneking system elucidates the concept of surgical margin and may provide the historic context for the development of metastasis-specific surgical concepts. The Enneking system recommends radical or wide margin en bloc resection in cases of primary high-grade malignant tumors. The goal of en bloc resection is to remove the tumor in one piece without entering the margin. Radical margin surgery requires the excision of the entire anatomic compartment that harbors the tumor. Wide margin resection preserves normal tissue around the entire tumor, whereas a marginal margin resection is carried through the reactive zone of the tumor. The residual reactive tissue after a marginal margin surgery may contain "satellite" tumor cells and both marginal and wide margin dissection cannot eliminate the risk of residual skip lesions. Thus, in the absence of radical margin, Enneking recommended adjuvant therapy in cases of high-grade malignant tumors in order to treat the skip lesions and minimize the risk of recurrence.[1,2]

The complex anatomy of the surrounding structures and the central location of the spinal cord within the spinal column present unique challenges to the application of the Enneking principles in the treatment of spinal tumors. The majority of spinal metastatic solid tumors originate from the osseous structures of the vertebrae, with the dorsal vertebral body being the most common tumor site.[3] The discussion of a single vertebra as an individual surgical compartment requires clear understanding of the surrounding tissues that may prevent tumor spread and that are the most likely routes of tumor spread outside of the vertebra.[4] The barrier tissues surrounding the vertebra include ligaments (anterior longitudinal ligament [ALL], posterior longitudinal ligament [PLL], ligamentum flavum, interspinous ligament, and supraspinous ligament), periosteum (lateral to the vertebral body, surrounding the spinal canal, and dorsal and lateral to the lamina and spinous process), and intervertebral disk (cartilaginous end plate, annulus fibrosus, and nucleus pulposus).

Examination of en bloc surgical specimens demonstrated the highest degree of tumor invasion in the PLL and lateral periosteum.[3] The ALL, ligamentum flavum, and intervertebral disk appeared to act as good barriers to tumor penetration. Further analysis of tumor spread pattern showed that the lateral PLL was the most likely route of vertical extension in metastatic tumors, followed by the central PLL. The strong longitudinal central attachment of the PLL compared with the thinner ligament laterally provides an explanation for this spread pattern. The presence of a fibrous reactive membrane was noted in several specimens even after extension outside of these anatomic barriers. The presence of such a capsule implies the possibility of a marginal margin resection according to the Enneking principles. However, the high likelihood of satellite microscopic disease outside of the capsule has to be considered in cases of malignant tumors, which includes all metastases.

In 1997, two systems aimed at translating the resection principles of the Enneking system into the spine-specific context were proposed. The Surgical Classification of the Vertebral Tumors developed by Tomita et al[5] (**Fig. 4.1**) and applicable to metastases, divides the tumors into intracompartmental (confined to the vertebra), extracompartmental (extraosseous extension), and multifocal skip lesions, and classifies them also based on the extent of dorsal extension along the vertebra (vertebral body only, extension into pedicle and then lamina). The Weinstein, Boriani, and Biagini (WBB) Surgical Staging System, applicable to primary spinal tumors, divides the axial plane of the vertebral body into 12 radial zones, similar to a clock face, and into five concentric zones, thereby providing a systematic description of the extent and location of the tumor around the spinal cord and its extraosseous extension[6] (**Fig. 4.2**). Both systems were developed in order to provide a common language when describing the location and extent of the tumor and to determine what type of surgical margin would be feasible. Although a radical margin, or resection of the entire spinal compartment, is not feasible, certain tumors may be amenable to wide or marginal margin resection.

■ Surgical Technique

Vertebrectomy, sagittal resection, and posterior arch resection represent the three main methods of en bloc resection in the spine.[6] Tumors centered in the vertebral body may be removed en bloc by carrying out a vertebrectomy or excision of the entire vertebral body.

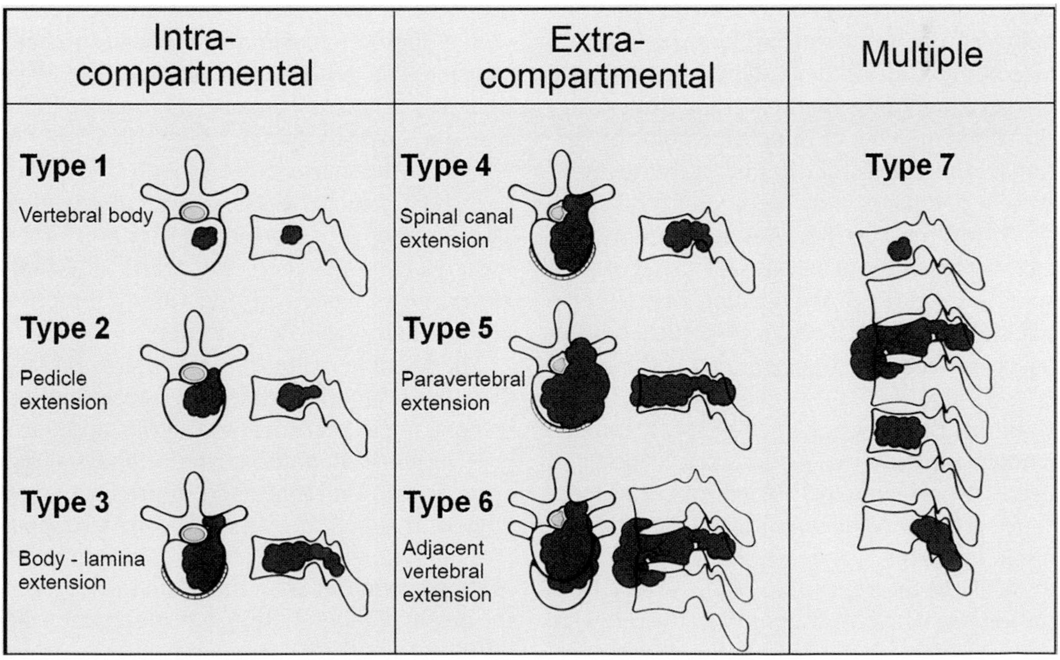

Intra-compartmental	Extra-compartmental	Multiple
Type 1 Vertebral body	**Type 4** Spinal canal extension	**Type 7**
Type 2 Pedicle extension	**Type 5** Paravertebral extension	
Type 3 Body - lamina extension	**Type 6** Adjacent vertebral extension	

Fig. 4.1 Tomita classification of vertebral tumors. (From Kawahara N, Tomita K, Murakami H, Demura S. Total en bloc spondylectomy for spinal tumors: surgical techniques and related basic background. Orthop Clin North Am 2009;40:47–63. Reproduced with permission from Elsevier.)

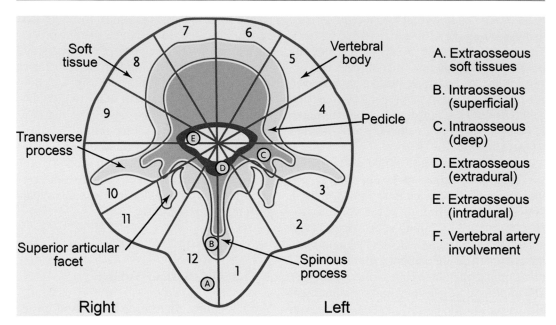

Fig. 4.2 Weinstein-Boriani-Biagini surgical staging system. (From Boriani S, Weinstein JN, Biagini R. Primary bone tumors of the spine. Terminology and surgical staging. Spine 1997;22:1036–1044. Reproduced with permission from Wolters Kluwer Health.)

Tumors arising from the pedicle, transverse process, or eccentrically located in the vertebral body may be removed en bloc using sagittal osteotomy through the posterior elements and the vertebral body. Tumors arising from posterior elements may be removed en bloc by sectioning the pedicles and removing the posterior arch in one piece.[2] Any method of total spondylectomy must include the opening of the spinal canal in order to permit safe passage of the spinal cord through the opening. Therefore, in cases of a tumor that begins to encircle the spinal cord, deliberate transgression of the tumor is likely required.

Prior to en bloc resection of spinal tumors, embolization may be undertaken in order to decrease intraoperative blood loss. Kawahara et al[7] recommend embolization of bilateral segmental arteries at the excision levels in order to facilitate the separation of the artery from the vertebral body and along with the cephalad and caudal levels. Such embolization may reduce blood loss in cases where intentional or unintentional tumor transgression takes place.

Embolization of three levels significantly reduced the intraoperative blood loss compared with embolization of only the level with tumor invasion. Preoperative embolization also helps to define segmental arteries that anastomose with the anterior spinal artery, including the artery of Adamkiewicz.[8] Although sacrifice of the artery of Adamkiewicz is generally avoided, Murakami et al[9] reported a series of 15 total spondylectomies where the artery of Adamkiewicz was ligated during tumor resection without neurologic deterioration.

The location of the tumor dictates the approach. En bloc resection can be carried out using a single posterior or anterior approach, or a combination of the posterior and anterior approaches. The combined approaches may be performed on the same day or as two separate operations. The extent of tumor invasion of the surrounding structures and the level and the extent of required spinal reconstruction determine the optimal combination of approaches. Generally, a combination of anterior and posterior approaches is required in order to perform an en bloc resection of lumbar tumors. When invasion of the major vessels, segmental arteries, and thoracic or abdominal organs is suspected, an anterior dissection may be performed during the first stage of the operation, followed by the posterior approach for the en bloc excision. The order of the anterior and posterior approaches has to be tailored to specific level and tumor anatomy and determined individually for each case.

The posterior approach should expose two or three levels above and below the tumor. Laterally, approximately 4 to 5 cm of the bilateral ribs or the entire transverse process must be exposed at the levels involved by tumor and at least one level adjacent to the tumor. Superiorly the spinous process and the inferior articulating processes of the level above the tumor and inferiorly the ligamentous attachment of the spinous process and the superior articulating processes of the level below the tumor must be sectioned in order to release the posterior elements of tumor. In the thoracic spine, the 3- to 4-cm segments of the ribs distal to the costovertebral junction are removed in order to expose the pedicles of the tumor level. The neurovascular bundle running along the inferior edge of the rib is identified and separated or sacrificed prior to removal of the rib. Periosteal dissection is carried out along the pars interarticularis and pedicles in order to allow a safe osteotomy through the pedicles.

Posterolateral pedicle fixation is carried out two or three levels above the excision. Only one rod is placed at this time, on the side opposite the direction of the rotation of the final en bloc specimen. Only temporary tightening of the screw rod construct should be carried out because distraction and compression maneuvers may be required. The osteotomy may be carried out using a thread-wire saw, an osteotome, or a drill. Once the pedicles are sectioned and the posterior elements are released from the levels above and below the tumor, the pedicle, transverse process, lamina, and spinous process complex of the levels involved by tumor may be removed in one piece.

Identification of the segmental artery at the level of the vertebrectomy is of paramount importance. This artery is usually located lateral to the pedicle. The spinal branch of the segmental artery must be identified and ligated. In the thoracic spine, the nerve roots can generally be safely sacrificed below T1, which eliminates the risk of evulsion and facilitates the circumferential exposure and dissection. The surrounding pleura or iliopsoas muscle are bluntly dissected off the vertebral body, with care being taken to control the segmental artery at all times. The bilateral segmental arteries are followed to the aorta, which is carefully dissected off the left ventral surface of the vertebral body. The segmental arteries are clipped, coagulated, and sectioned in order to prevent evulsion of these arteries off the aorta. This dissection is completed in the cephalocaudal direction until all of the vertebral bodies that will be removed en bloc are separated from the surrounding lateral and ventral structures. Malleable retractors are used to maintain the separation and to protect the paraspinal structures.

The vertebrae involved by tumor are generally separated from the remaining spinal column at the cephalad and caudal disk spaces. This can be carried out using a thread-wire saw or osteotomes.[7,8] Various devices have been developed to facilitate this step. If a lateral direction of the cut is chosen, the surgeon must remember the concave shape of the dorsal surface of the vertebral body and create a safe channel for the saw prior to stretching it in order to avoid dural damage. The anterior and posterior longitudinal ligaments must also be sectioned in order to complete the release of the tumor, and the epidural venous plexus dorsal to the PLL must be fully coagulated in order to minimize the bleeding. Finally, the ventral dural surface must be separated from the vertebrectomy segment and Hoffman's ligaments must be carefully sectioned. This can be carried out through blunt dissection using angled dissectors. At this point the vertebrectomy specimen is entirely mobilized and can be rotated around the spinal cord in order to complete the removal. Anterior column reconstruction is completed using a distractible or mesh titanium cage; alternatively, a distractible polyetheretherketone (PEEK) cage may be used.

Axial loading of the anterior construct is en-sured with compression of the posterolateral instrumentation. Autologous rib graft may be used to maximize the chances of osseous fusion during the reconstruction of the anterior and posterior columns. Irrigation of the resection cavity with distilled water and high-concen-tration cisplatinum can be performed to locally treat microscopic residual tumor.

If anterior release of the tumor from vital thoracic or abdominal structures is required prior to the posterior approach, a thoracotomy may be used or a retroperitoneal approach to L2-L4 and a transperitoneal approach to the L5 level. An approach surgeon may be consulted, depending on the preference and experience of the surgeon and institutional practice. These procedures can be carried out using traditional open techniques or a mini-open or thoraco-scopic approach.[10] Thoracoscopy provides a minimally invasive alternative to ventral liga-tion of the segmental arteries and does not require a postoperative chest tube.[11] The com-bined posterior-anterior approach may be car-ried out with the patient placed in the lateral position.[12]

■ Local Control

En bloc excision of spinal metastases provides excellent neurologic outcomes and reliable local tumor control (**Fig. 4.3**), with only a few recur-rences reported (**Table 4.1**). Murakami et al[13] examined the neurologic function after tho-racic en bloc tumor resection in 79 patients, with 53 of these patients undergoing surgery for metastatic tumors. Within the entire group, 46 patients had a neurologic deficit, and 25 of them experienced an improvement of at least one Frankel grade, whereas the remaining pa-tients experienced an improvement in neuro-logic symptoms even if it did not translate into a full Frankel grade improvement.

Tomita et al[5] reported no recurrences in 20 patients who underwent en bloc resection for a variety of metastatic tumor histologies. The

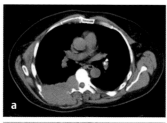
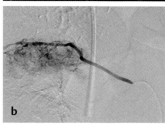
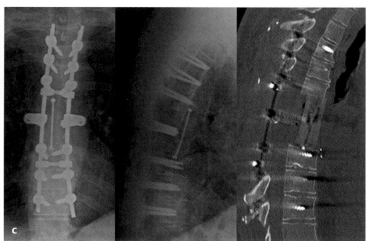

Fig. 4.3a–c Case example of a 58-year-old man with **(a)** solitary renal metastasis to the T6 and T7 levels with chest wall invasion on the right. **(b)** The patient underwent preoperative embolization of the tumor followed by T6 and T7 spondylectomy with right-sided chest wall resection for en bloc tumor resection. **(c)** The stabilization was carried out using pedicle fixation three levels above and below the tumor, and carbon fiber cage and allograft recon-struction of the anterior column. Adjuvant conven-tional external beam radiation was administered. His most recent follow-up, 3 years and 3 months after surgery, shows no evidence of local recurrence and no evidence of systemic disease. (Courtesy of Jean-Paul Wolinsky, MD, Johns Hopkins University.)

Table 4.1 Summary of Publications Describing the Outcome of Spondylectomy for En Bloc Resection of Metastases in at Least 10 Patients

Study	Number of Patients	Recurrence	EBL (cc)	Surgical Time (Hours)	Complications
Tomita et al (1994)	20	0	1,650	7.8	10% major
Fourney et al (2001)	15	0	2,100	10.6	27% major
Sakaura et al (2004)	12	17%	1,925	7.3	N/A
Melcher et al (2007)	12	0	15 PRBC, 20 FFP	9.2	1 infection, 1 wound
Li et al (2009)	32	3%	1,536	7.7	18.75% major, 9.4 % minor
Demura et al (2011)	10	10%	1,713	9.1	2 pleural effusion, 1 chylothorax
Fang et al (2012)	17	0	1,720	6.7	12%
Huang et al (2013)	14	0	2,300	7.2	N/A

Abbreviations: EBL, estimated blood loss; FFP, fresh frozen plasma; N/A, not available; PRBC, packed red blood cells.

median follow-up in this group was 9 months, with nine patients alive at the completion of the analysis and a range of 8- to 30-month follow-up among survivors. Fifteen metastatic tumors, mostly metastatic renal cell carcinoma, were resected using a simultaneous anterior-posterior approach with the patient placed in the lateral position. No recurrences were observed after a median follow-up of 6 months, with two patients surviving over 2 years without local recurrence. Sakaura et al[14] reported the outcome of en bloc resection in 12 patients, mostly with metastatic breast, thyroid, and renal cell carcinoma metastases. The overall survival was 58%, with median follow-up of 61 months in survivors and 23 months in patients who died. The authors observed two local recurrences 25 months after surgery, both in patients with tumors with paraspinal extension. Eight patients had tumor progression at other sites at a median of 5 months after surgery.

Melcher et al[11] performed en bloc resection on 12 patients with solitary metastases, with median survival of 29 months. No local recurrences were observed with follow-up ranging from 2 to 75 months. Four patients developed distant metastases at an average of 5.3 months, with two of these patients dying. Of note, eight patients were reported to have no evidence of disease. Li et al[15] reported the outcome of en bloc resection in 32 patients with spinal metastases, with most of the tumors originating in the kidney. Twenty-six of the patients underwent a vertebrectomy, three underwent a sagittal resection, and three had a posterior resection. The median survival was 40.1 months (range, 16–66 months) with only one patient having a local recurrence. Fang et al[10] performed en bloc resection in 17 patients with spinal metastatic tumors with an average follow-up of 15.3 months. No recurrences were observed, with 59% of the patients dying with an average survival of 12 months. Finally, Huang et al[8] performed en bloc resection in 14 patients, with no evidence of local recurrence. The mean follow-up was 14 months (range, 3–23 months), with five patients dying during the study period.

Several patient series report the results of en bloc resection in patients with specific histologies. Demura et al[16] and Matsumoto[17] examined the results of en bloc resection in patients with metastatic thyroid carcinoma. Demura et al treated six patients with follicular, three with papillary, and one with medullary thyroid carcinoma with median follow-up of 54 months. They reported one local recurrence at about 3 years after surgery. Three patients died of disease, five are alive with disease, and two have no evidence of disease. The 5-year survival in this group was 90%. Matsumoto et al performed en bloc resection in six patients with follicular and two with papillary thyroid carcinoma. Two patients experienced local recurrence 3.3 and 8 years after surgery, with one of the patients undergoing intralesional resection of the recurrence. All of the patients in this series were alive with a mean follow-up of 6.4 years, and five patients had no evidence of disease.

Murakami et al[18] reported the results of en bloc resection in six patients with metastatic lung adenocarcinoma. Four surviving patients were followed for an average of 46 months without evidence of local recurrence. Several case reports describe long-term local control after en bloc resection of metastatic paraganglioma, pheochromocytoma, and myxoid liposarcoma.

■ Complications

En bloc excision of spinal tumors is a challenging operation that may be associated with significant intraoperative and early and late postoperative morbidity. The reported average operative times range between 6.7 and 10.6 hours, with major series reporting a mean estimated blood loss ranging from 1.5 to 2.3 L[5,8,10–12,14,15] (**Table 4.1**). The reported complication rates range from 10 to 27%. Boriani et al[19] critically examined the morbidity of en bloc spinal surgery in 134 patients, 44 of whom had metastatic tumors. The complications were classified as minor and major, with complications that significantly affected the expected postoperative recovery course classified as "major." The authors reported 70 complications in 47 patients (35.1%). A total of 41 major complications occurred in 26 patients, including vena cava and aortic injuries, massive intraoperative hemorrhage, myocardial infarction, pulmonary embolism, renal failure, subdural hematoma, paraplegia due to postoperative hematoma, deep wound infections, and posterior instrumentation revision. Three deaths (2%) occurred due to the surgical complications. Minor complications included durotomies,

minor vascular injury, asymptomatic deformity, retrograde ejaculation, and acute renal failure. The use of combined surgical approaches was associated with increased risk of minor and major complications, and the risk of major complications increased with the number of resection levels.

■ Indications

The treatment goals of spinal metastases include local control, preservation, and restoration of neurologic function and spinal stability and pain control. These goals are accomplished using various combinations of surgery, radiation, and chemotherapy. Surgical indications include stabilization of a mechanically unstable spinal column, decompression of the neural elements, and optimization of local tumor control. The prospective study conducted by Patchell et al[20] found that in patients with spinal cord compression secondary to solid metastatic tumors surgery followed by radiation therapy provides superior functional outcomes compared with radiation therapy alone. However, in this study patients underwent a broad range of operative interventions, which precludes any conclusions about the optimal surgical method. To date, a randomized study comparing various types of surgery has not been conducted. The available retrospective studies are difficult to compare due to a great variety of chemotherapy and radiation options available in the neoadjuvant and adjuvant settings, and due to the extremely heterogeneous patient population.

Surgeons have developed several scoring systems and decision frameworks to help guide decision making in patients with metastatic spine tumors. The Tokuhashi and Tomita scoring systems focus on the expected survival in order to guide surgical strategy.[21,22] The Tomita scoring system looks at the primary tumor histology, the extent of visceral metastases, and the number of osseous metastases in order to determine the treatment goal.[22] The treatment goal categories include long-, middle-, and short-term palliation, and terminal care. For patients with the goal of long-term palliation, wide or marginal excision is recommended, and for patients with the goal of middle-term palliation, marginal or intralesional excision is recommended. Among the 28 patients for whom, according to their scoring system, long- or middle-term palliation was recommended and who underwent en bloc excision with a wide or marginal margin, 26 had no evidence of local recurrence, with an average survival of 38.2 months.

The Tokuhashi scoring system considers the performance status, number of spinal and extraspinal bone metastases, extent of visceral metastases, primary tumor histology, and the neurologic status in order to divide the patients into groups with expected survival of less than 6 months, between 6 months and 1 year, and longer than 1 year.[21] Based on these survival categories, conservative treatment, palliative surgery, or excisional surgery is recommended. However, only 22 out of 246 patients who were included in the analysis had scores that qualified them for excisional surgery and only five of them underwent en bloc excision. Although both of these scoring systems capture some of the vital considerations in predicting the patients' expected survival, they omit the consideration of systemic and radiation therapy as treatment options for spinal metastases, placing great emphasis on surgery.

The treatment algorithm implemented by Gasbarrini et al[23] takes the sensitivity of the tumor to radiation therapy, chemotherapy, hormonal therapy, and immunotherapy into consideration in order to guide the treatment of spinal metastases. They recommend that patients with metastases that are resistant to radiation and systemic therapy undergo excisional surgery, with en bloc resection suggested for patients with isolated metastases and debulking surgery suggested for patients with multiple metastases. Thus, in this algorithm, the decision to undergo surgery largely hinges on the sensitivity of the tumor to radiation and systemic therapy, with en bloc resection recommended for patients whose tumors cannot effectively be controlled with radiation or systemic therapy.

During the past decade the concept of radiation sensitivity of tumors has undergone a dramatic change with implementation of stereotactic radiosurgery (SRS). The majority of solid tumor metastases, with the exception of breast and prostate histology, are resistant to conventionally fractionated radiation, which has been available for decades and has served as the determinant of tumor sensitivity to radiation.[24] However, spinal SRS overcomes this resistance in the majority of cases, providing effective local tumor control even in tumors that exhibit resistance to conventional external beam radiation therapy (cEBRT). SRS may be safely employed as the single-treatment option in patients who do not require surgical stabilization or decompression or as a postoperative adjuvant. It can also be administered in previously radiated tumors in cases of recurrence. In a series of 500 patients treated with radiosurgery, Gerszten et al[25] reported radiographic control in 88% of the tumors with a median follow-up of 21 months. Garg et al[26] also reported an actuarial 18-month local tumor control of 88% in 63 tumors treated with single-fraction SRS. Furthermore, tumor control has been shown to be dose dependent, and the risk of local radiographic tumor progression after high-dose single-fraction radiation (24 Gy) was estimated to be 4% with 3-year follow-up.[27] Finally, when SRS was used as the primary form of tumor control in patients who underwent circumferential decompression of the spinal cord and resection of the epidural tumor extension without resection of the tumor-infiltrated vertebral body or paraspinal tumor, the risk of local tumor progression at 1 year after treatment was 9% after single-fraction radiotherapy and 4% after high-dose hypofractionated radiotherapy.[28] The neurologic, oncological, mechanical, and systemic (NOMS) paradigm integrates spinal SRS into the decision-making process, placing greater emphasis on the role of radiotherapy in local tumor control while recommending surgery for patients who require stabilization or spinal cord decompression.[29]

Local tumor control for the duration of the patient's life represents one of the primary goals of treatment of spinal metastases. The survival prediction can often present a challenge, especially with the rapid evolution of systemic therapy options. Although several scoring systems facilitate this estimation by highlighting the primary considerations, each treatment decision must be tailored to the modern therapeutic options and patient-specific medical and social factors. In the overwhelming majority of patients with spinal metastases, treatment goals remain palliative and must be made in the context of expected survival ranging from a few months to a few years and the importance of expedient continuation or commencement of systemic therapy. Thus, the penalty of postoperative complication may be devastating if it leads to delay in systemic therapy and if disease progression cannot be controlled, and the risk of complication must be weighed against the benefit of local tumor control.

The reported local recurrence rates after en bloc excision of spinal metastases are extremely low, with only three recurrences (2%) reported among the 122 patients studied in the seven series that include more than 10 patients.[5,8,10–12,14,15] The long follow-up reported for some of the series emphasizes the importance of careful patient selection for this operation. However, the variability of follow-up methods for assessing tumor recurrence and the retrospective nature of most studies limit the strength of evidence presented by the surgical series. Furthermore, these operations are challenging, and a complication rate as high as 35% has been reported even from one of the world's leading centers in en bloc spinal tumor excision.

The potential for significant hemodynamic stress during surgery even after embolization and the long-term survival requirement in order to justify en bloc excision exclude the majority of patients with metastatic cancer. The reliable local control provided by high-dose SRS provides a low-morbidity alternative to en bloc excision and has gained prominence as more medical centers integrate spinal radiosurgery into their treatment paradigms. Review of treatment results in patients with solitary renal metastases after SRS compared with en bloc resection showed comparable local control.[30] Although the strength of the recommendation was limited by the quality of available evidence, SRS was recommended as first-line treatment in patients with solitary spinal renal metastases and no or minimal epidural tumor extension. Currently, this recommendation can be extended to most metastases, based on accumulating data describing histology-independent durable control provided by SRS.

In most cases without spinal cord compression, en bloc resection can be reserved for tumors that progress in spite of previous optimal radiation therapy. On the other hand, in patients with spinal cord compression by solid tumors, surgery followed by radiation therapy continues to be the recommended treatment. In these cases and in carefully selected patients, en bloc resection may provide effective local tumor control; however, intralesional resection of the epidural tumor component with circumferential spinal cord decompression provides a less invasive alternative and has been shown to also provide effective local tumor control when followed by high-dose radiation therapy.[28]

■ Chapter Summary

Local tumor control represents one of the primary goals in the treatment of spinal metastases. The importance of tumor margin preservation and wide margin excision was shown in patients with primary musculoskeletal tumors and subsequently incorporated into some of the treatment systems for spinal metastases.[5,6] The technique of spinal en bloc resection generally requires a circumferential dissection around the vertebral column without violating the tumor margin, followed by instrumented stabilization.[7] Depending on the level and the degree of paraspinal extension, anterior, posterior, or combined approaches may be required. The local control rates after en bloc tumor resection have been outstanding, whereas some series report a high risk of perioperative complications. In the metastatic spine tumor patient population the risk of complication must be weighed against the importance of long-term tumor control in the setting of generally limited survival. Although a select patient population with long expected survival may be considered for en bloc tumor excision, spinal SRS provides an effective alternative to aggressive tumor resection in most patients while avoiding the potential morbidity of extensive surgery.

- Spinal SRS can provide comparable local control to en bloc resection with a significantly lower complication risk and therefore may represent a better option for tumor control.

Pearls

- The Weinstein-Boriani-Biagini Surgical Staging System and the Tomita Surgical Classification of the Vertebral Tumors can be used to describe the location and intra- and extraosseous extension of spinal tumors.
- En bloc resection options include vertebrectomy, sagittal resection, posterior arch resection, and spondylectomy for en bloc resection of tumor.
- Preoperative embolization decreases intraoperative blood loss during intralesional surgery.
- Segmental arteries must be carefully dissected and ligated.
- En bloc tumor excision provides durable local control in carefully selected patients.

Pitfalls

- Careful examination of ventral epidural space is mandatory because the most common route of tumor spread is between the PLL and the vertebral body.
- Hoffman's ligaments must be ligated in order to separate the en bloc specimen from the dura.
- The concave shape of the dorsal aspect of the vertebral body and the dural convexity at their interface must be taken into consideration when performing the osteotomy in the dorsal third of the vertebral body or intervertebral disk space.

References

Five Must-Read References

1. Enneking WF, Spanier SS, Goodman MA. A system for the surgical staging of musculoskeletal sarcoma. Clin Orthop Relat Res 1980;153:106–120
2. Enneking WF. A system of staging musculoskeletal neoplasms. Clin Orthop Relat Res 1986;204:9–24
3. Sasagawa T, Kawahara N, Murakami H, et al. The route of metastatic vertebral tumors extending to the adjacent vertebral body: a histological study. J Orthop Sci 2011;16:203–211
4. Fujita T, Ueda Y, Kawahara N, Baba H, Tomita K. Local spread of metastatic vertebral tumors. A histologic study. Spine 1997;22:1905–1912
5. Tomita K, Kawahara N, Baba H, Tsuchiya H, Nagata S, Toribatake Y. Total en bloc spondylectomy for solitary spinal metastases. Int Orthop 1994;18:291–298
6. Boriani S, Weinstein JN, Biagini R. Primary bone tumors of the spine. Terminology and surgical staging. Spine 1997;22:1036–1044
7. Kawahara N, Tomita K, Murakami H, Demura S. Total en bloc spondylectomy for spinal tumors: surgical techniques and related basic background. Orthop Clin North Am 2009;40:47–63, vi
8. Huang L, Chen K, Ye JC, et al. Modified total en bloc spondylectomy for thoracolumbar spinal tumors via a single posterior approach. Eur Spine J 2013;22:556–564
9. Murakami H, Kawahara N, Tomita K, Demura S, Kato S, Yoshioka K. Does interruption of the artery of Adamkiewicz during total en bloc spondylectomy affect neurologic function? Spine 2010;35:E1187–E1192

10. Fang T, Dong J, Zhou X, McGuire RA Jr, Li X. Comparison of mini-open anterior corpectomy and posterior total en bloc spondylectomy for solitary metastases of the thoracolumbar spine. J Neurosurg Spine 2012;17:271–279
11. Melcher I, Disch AC, Khodadadyan-Klostermann C, et al. Primary malignant bone tumors and solitary metastases of the thoracolumbar spine: results by management with total en bloc spondylectomy. Eur Spine J 2007;16:1193–1202
12. Fourney DR, Abi-Said D, Rhines LD, et al. Simultaneous anterior-posterior approach to the thoracic and lumbar spine for the radical resection of tumors followed by reconstruction and stabilization. J Neurosurg 2001;94(2, Suppl):232–244
13. Murakami H, Kawahara N, Demura S, Kato S, Yoshioka K, Tomita K. Neurological function after total en bloc spondylectomy for thoracic spinal tumors. J Neurosurg Spine 2010;12:253–256
14. Sakaura H, Hosono N, Mukai Y, Ishii T, Yonenobu K, Yoshikawa H. Outcome of total en bloc spondylectomy for solitary metastasis of the thoracolumbar spine. J Spinal Disord Tech 2004;17:297–300
15. Li H, Gasbarrini A, Cappuccio M, et al. Outcome of excisional surgeries for the patients with spinal metastases. Eur Spine J 2009;18:1423–1430
16. Demura S, Kawahara N, Murakami H, et al. Total en bloc spondylectomy for spinal metastases in thyroid carcinoma. J Neurosurg Spine 2011;14:172–176
17. Matsumoto M. Total en bloc spondylectomy for spinal metastasis of differentiated thyroid cancers: a

long-term follow-up. J Spinal Disord Tech 2012; 10/17:1

18. Murakami H, Kawahara N, Demura S, Kato S, Yoshioka K, Tomita K. Total en bloc spondylectomy for lung cancer metastasis to the spine. J Neurosurg Spine 2010;13:414–417

19. Boriani S, Bandiera S, Donthineni R, et al. Morbidity of en bloc resections in the spine. Eur Spine J 2010; 19:231–241

20. Patchell RA, Tibbs PA, Regine WF, et al. Direct decompressive surgical resection in the treatment of spinal cord compression caused by metastatic cancer: a randomised trial. Lancet 2005;366:643–648

21. Tokuhashi Y, Matsuzaki H, Oda H, Oshima M, Ryu J. A revised scoring system for preoperative evaluation of metastatic spine tumor prognosis. Spine 2005;30: 2186–2191

22. Tomita K, Kawahara N, Kobayashi T, Yoshida A, Murakami H, Akamaru T. Surgical strategy for spinal metastases. Spine 2001;26:298–306

23. Gasbarrini A, Li H, Cappuccio M, et al. Efficacy evaluation of a new treatment algorithm for spinal metastases. Spine 2010;35:1466–1470

24. Gerszten PC, Mendel E, Yamada Y. Radiotherapy and radiosurgery for metastatic spine disease: what are the options, indications, and outcomes? Spine 2009; 34(22, Suppl):S78–S92

25. Gerszten PC, Burton SA, Ozhasoglu C, Welch WC. Radiosurgery for spinal metastases: clinical experience in 500 cases from a single institution. Spine 2007; 32:193–199

26. Garg AK, Shiu AS, Yang J, et al. Phase 1/2 trial of single-session stereotactic body radiotherapy for previously unirradiated spinal metastases. Cancer 2012; 118:5069–5077

27. Yamada Y, Cox BW, Zelefsky MJ, et al. An analysis of prognostic factors for local control of malignant spine tumors treated with spine radiosurgery. Paper presented at the International Journal of Radiation Oncology, Biology, Physics, October 1, 2011

28. Laufer I, Iorgulescu JB, Chapman T, et al. Local disease control for spinal metastases following "separation surgery" and adjuvant hypofractionated or high-dose single-fraction stereotactic radiosurgery: outcome analysis in 186 patients. J Neurosurg Spine 2013;18: 207–214

29. Laufer I, Rubin DG, Lis E, et al. The NOMS framework: approach to the treatment of spinal metastatic tumors. Oncologist 2013;18:744–751

30. Bilsky MH, Laufer I, Burch S. Shifting paradigms in the treatment of metastatic spine disease. Spine 2009; 34(22, Suppl):S101–S107

5

Region-Specific Approaches

Ioan Adrian Lina, Patricia L. Zadnik, and Daniel M. Sciubba

■ Introduction

The spine is the third most common location of secondary metastases, after the lung and liver, occurring in up to one third of all metastatic cancer patients.[1] Further, in a review of autopsy studies, it was reported that up to 70% of cancer patients had evidence of metastatic disease in the spinal column at the time of death.[2] Anatomically, an overwhelming majority of spinal metastases originate from the vertebral body rather than from the posterior elements.[3]

Patients with symptomatic spinal metastases most commonly present with pain or neurologic dysfunction. A systemic workup with a computed tomography (CT) scan of the chest, abdomen, and pelvis for cancer staging may be necessary to guide surgical decision making, and in patients without a known primary tumor, a fine-needle biopsy under CT guidance should be performed. Patients with metastatic epidural spinal cord compression should be given high-dose dexamethasone, and in patients who respond to this therapy, radiation will likely provide relief.[4] Tumor pathology dictates the appropriateness of adjuvant therapy, as radiosensitive tumors such as small-cell lung carcinoma, lymphoma, and multiple myeloma rarely require open decompression, as radiation alone provides effective palliation for patients at the end of life. Intermediately radiosensitive tumors include breast and prostate cancer, whereas melanoma is relatively radioresistant.

For highly vascularized tumors, such as renal carcinoma, a preoperative angiogram with embolization should be considered to reduce the risk of intraoperative tumor bleeding during resection.[5] In all pathologies, surgery with radiation should be considered if the patient is expected to live for longer than 3 months.[6] In the landmark randomized controlled clinical trial of radiation alone versus radiation with surgery, Patchell and colleagues[7] found that patient survival increased and the use of morphine and corticosteroids decreased with radiation and surgery compared with surgery alone.

Several scoring systems help to guide surgical decision making. The Tokuhashi score has been used to identify if an excision or palliative strategy should be offered.[8] Treatment goals can be tailored to the patient's visceral and bony disease burden and grade of the malignancy as proposed in the Tomita score.[9] The Spinal Instability Neoplastic Score (SINS) was proposed by the Spine Oncology Study Group (SOSG) to incorporate multiple variables to determine the stability, pending instability or gross instability caused by a primary or metastatic lesion in the spine.[10]

Complex approaches requiring prolonged recovery times are contraindicated if the life expectancy of the patient does not exceed 3 months, and radiation therapy may be offered for palliative treatment of pain.[6] For patients with widespread metastases in the spinal column, direct decompressive surgery (i.e., laminectomy) with adjuvant radiotherapy improves neurologic outcomes and reduces the need for steroids and opioid analgesics.[7] It should also be taken into account that surgical intervention delays radiation treatment due to the additional time needed for wound healing. En bloc resection for metastatic disease has been debated in the literature. Oncological cure is unlikely for metastatic disease, as widespread microscopic tumor foci are likely present; however, patients may survive many years beyond surgery. In a systemic review of the literature, Cloyd and colleagues[11] found 5-year survival rates of 37.5% for patients undergoing en bloc spondylectomy for metastatic cancer in the spinal column. Aside from the technical demand of the surgery, the major risks of en bloc resection include nerve damage, excessive bleeding, spinal cord ischemia or stroke, and tumor spillage with disruption of the capsule or intralesional curettage. When planning en bloc resection, the patient must be consulted to determine his or her preferences and goals of care.

This chapter reviews the approaches used for surgical resection of metastatic tumors in specific regions of the spine (**Fig. 5.1**), and describes patient positioning and approaches as well as the common complications associated with each surgical intervention. Complications are summarized in **Table 5.1**.

■ Cervical Spine

The cervical spine comprises only 10 to 20% of metastatic spine disease cases; however, instability due to cervical metastases can lead to profound morbidity.[12] More than 90% of patients with metastatic disease in the cervical spine present with nonmechanical neck pain as their chief complaint.[13] Patients may also report referred pain in the shoulders. Biomechanically, in the subaxial spine, lytic invasion of metastatic tumor in the cancellous bone of the vertebral body increases the risk of collapse and subsequent loss of lordosis. At the atlantoaxial level, involvement of the C1 lateral mass leads to pain on rotational head movements. Stability of the atlantoaxial ligamentous complex, particularly the transverse ligament, determines the stability of the C1/C2 vertebral bodies. The wider spinal canal in the atlantoaxial spine reduces the risk of metastatic epidural spinal cord compression, and as a result anterior atlantoaxial subluxation is a more common cause of canal stenosis at this level.[14] Lateral flexion-extension radiographs of the spine can help identify the degree of spondylolisthesis and ultimately identify regions of instability in the cervical spine.

When assessing a patient with a cervical metastasis, take a thorough history and perform a physical examination to confirm the patient's chief complaint. Cervical myelopathy, characterized by weakness in the hands and relative preservation of lower extremity function, may be the result of degenerative disease in the cervical spine unrelated to the metastatic process. Although vertebral body involvement from a metastatic lesion may be the most radiographically impressive element of the patient's imaging, it may not be the sole cause of the neurologic impairment. Loss of cervical lordosis, degenerative disk disease with multilevel stenosis, or congenital stenosis may be the main cause of a patient's symptoms and should be considered when planning surgery. In patients with a loss of lordosis, posterior reduction and fixation alone will not restore anatomic alignment, and an anterior approach is recommended.

Posterior Approach

Posterior laminectomy or hemilaminectomy with instrumented fixation is frequently used for patients with preserved cervical lordosis suffering from metastatic disease in the cervical spine. Although the posterior elements are rarely involved in metastatic cervical tumors, decompressive laminectomy or foraminotomy are less invasive surgical procedures to provide relief of myelopathy or cervical radiculopathy. Instrumented fusion reduces the pain associated with subluxation and instability. Bone quality should also be taken into consideration in order to assess the patient's risk of instrumentation failure, and cement can be used to reinforce screw purchase.

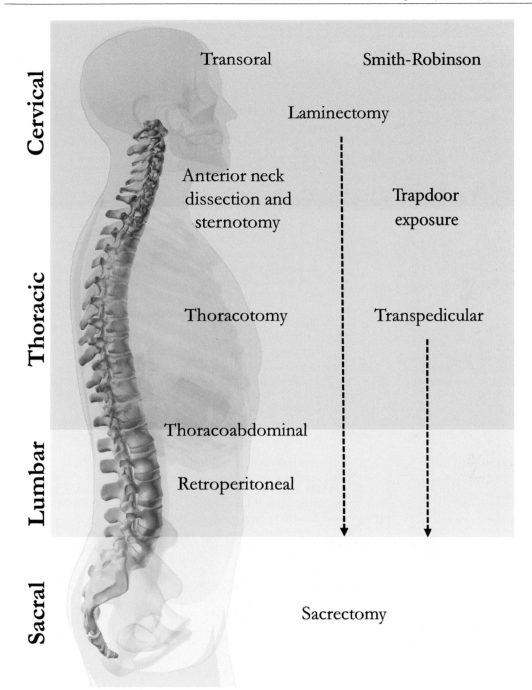

Fig. 5.1 Schematic depicting region-specific approaches to the spine for resection of metastatic tumors. Approaches between regions are effective for cross-junctional access. *Black dashed arrows* demonstrate approaches commonly used at multiple regions.

Table 5.1 Complications Associated with Each Surgical Intervention

Approach	Spinal Levels	Advantages	Complications
Laminectomy	All levels	• Well known to spinal surgeons • Low risk of complications	• Risk of vertebral artery injury • Cannot reduce anterior cord compression • Complications from improper screw placement
Transoral	C0-C3	• Anterior access to upper cervical spine	• High learning curve • Extensive recovery time • High prevalence of comorbidities
Smith-Robinson	C3-T1	• Generous exposure • Multilevel access	• Risk of esophageal and tracheal injury • Postoperative edema may necessitate tracheostomy
Anterior neck dissection and sternotomy	C4-T3	• Access to the cervicothoracic transition zone	• Risk of pulmonary injury and damage to the great vessels • Surgically challenging
Trapdoor exposure	T3-T4	• Optimal surgical window for accessing anterior pathologies	• Risk of hemopericardium and pulmonary injury • Violation of the thoracic cavity
Transpedicular	T1-L5	• Circumferential decompression posteriorly	• Interbody cage placement may necessitate nerve root ligation • Limited operative field • Higher risk of durotomy and CSF leaks
Thoracotomy	T5-T11	• Superior visualization of vertebral elements • Minimizes spinal cord manipulation	• Risk of pneumo- and hemothorax • Air leaks, pulmonary complications such as atelectasis
Thoracoabdominal	T11-L1	• Access to the thoracolumbar transition zone	• Diaphragm is incised circumferentially • Risk of injury to the spleen (left side) and kidney
Retroperitoneal	L1-L5	• Minimal violation of critical structures	• Risk of injury to the ureter and genitofemoral nerve

The patient is placed prone on the operating table with the head in a Mayfield fixator. A midline incision is made to provide adequate exposure of the level of interest. The paraspinal musculature is divided, and subperiosteal dissection facilitates direct visualization of the lamina. Although the C1 and C2 nerve roots can be sacrificed safely, subsequent nerve root damage to C3-C7 results in significant patient morbidity and should always be considered when weighing treatment options. Lateral mass screws may be used from C3 to C6, along with a fitted rod to mimic natural cervical lordosis. Intractable subluxations can warrant the placement of occipitocervical fusion (OCF) hardware, which requires a more extensive exposure and is beyond the scope of this chapter.

One of the primary risks associated with surgical intervention in the cervical spine is vertebral artery (VA) injury. Wright and Lauryssen[14] found that 4.1% of a cohort of 1,318 patients receiving transarticular screws incurred VA injury. Patients with tumor in this region or a history of radiation to the area may have distorted anatomy or scar tissue, further increasing the risk of vertebral artery injury. As a result, a preoperative three-dimensional (3D) CT angiogram should be considered prior to placing instrumentation in the craniovertebral junction. If a VA is injured intraoperatively, recall that the lateral mass screw acts to tamponade the vessel. Avoid removing the screw in the VA and do not place the contralateral screw, as bilateral VA injury will lead to devastating neurologic consequences. Perform an angiography immediately, if possible, to assess if endovascular repair via balloon occlusion, coil embolization, or stent deployment is feasible and to assess the patency of the contralateral VA.

Transoral Approach

The transoral approach allows visualization of the anterior aspect of C1-C3 with 15 to 20 mm of lateral exposure from the midline.[15] It is uncommonly performed in metastatic tumor patients, yet may be indicated for patients with significant anterior compression of the spinal cord involving the upper cervical vertebrae. For this approach, the patient is positioned supine with the neck in 10 to 15 degrees of extension in a three-point Mayfield headholder. Intraoperative fluoroscopy with a C-arm is recommended for localization. A preoperative lateral radiograph of the hyperextended neck is recommended to evaluate instability at the craniocervical junction that may be aggravated with patient positioning. Preoperative and intraoperative antibiotics should be given to cover anaerobes and oral flora. Intubation via an awake fiberoptic endotracheal intubation may be used or tracheostomy to provide ventilation without disrupting the operative field.

If necessary, the soft palate can be split at the midline to increase the operative field. Although greater extension of the surgical field is possible via maxillary osteotomy or mandibulotomy approaches, they should be used with extreme caution in metastatic tumor patients due to prolonged patient recovery times and

the high risk of complications. Posterior fixation is highly recommended following the transoral approach due to an increase in mechanical instability caused by the possible disruption of the alar, transverse, and anterior longitudinal ligaments.[16] As a result, treatment of the atlantoaxial spine often results in OCF; however, if the occipitoaxial joint remains stable, a limited C1-C2 fixation should be considered to preserve motion.[17]

The most common complications associated with the transoral approach include injury to the hypoglossal and lingual nerves with subsequent speech and swallowing difficulties. A nasogastric tube may be placed intraoperatively, or a percutaneous endoscopic gastrostomy (PEG) may be placed to provide adequate nutrition for the patient in the immediate postoperative period. As with most spinal surgeries, cerebrospinal fluid (CSF) leak secondary to incidental durotomy can lead to devastating complications and should be managed with a direct repair when possible, or a CSF diverting lumbar drain or shunt as necessary. Patients with CSF leak may complain of headaches, and are at risk of meningitis.[16] The splitting of the soft palate is also known to cause velopalatine incompetence, or the inability to completely close the soft palate resulting in nasal regurgitation of liquids during swallowing.[18]

Smith Robinson/Anterolateral Approach

First described by Smith and Robinson,[19] the anterolateral approach to the cervical spine enables anterior access to C3-T1. On the right side, the recurrent laryngeal nerve crosses medially at C6/C7, thus a left-sided approach is recommended at this level. For this approach, the head of the bead is elevated 30 degrees and the patient is positioned supine with the head fixed in a Mayfield clamp and rotated away from the incision, with a towel placed transversely under the scapula to allow for neck extension. The head is rotated about 15 degrees to the contralateral side. Nasotracheal intubation allows complete closure of the mandible and improves the exposure. A 3- to 5-cm incision is made along the midline to the posterior

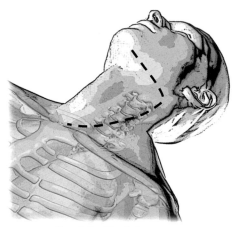

a Smith-Robinson

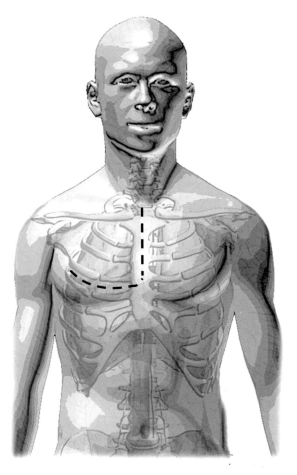

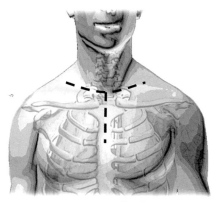

b Anterior neck dissection
and sternotomy

c Trapdoor

Fig. 5.2a–c Surgical markings for various approaches. **(a)** A "hockey stick" incision for the anterolateral (Smith-Robinson) approach to the subaxial cervical spine. **(b)** Anterior neck dissection and sternotomy approach with a T-shaped incision. **(c)** The trapdoor approach, which extends into the fourth interspace, allowing for retraction of the chest wall.

sternocleidomastoid for adequate exposure of two or three disk levels corresponding to the relevant pathology (**Fig. 5.2a**). The platysma is then divided at the anterior border of the sternocleidomastoid. Deep dissection proceeds with division of the pretracheal fascia to open the plane between the carotid sheath and the trachea and esophagus. Care should be taken to ensure the protection of the trachea, esophagus, and recurrent laryngeal nerve during dissection. Once adequate exposure is obtained, anterior corpectomy and resection can be per-

formed followed by the placement of a cage with allograft and anterior plate fixation. Concomitant posterior fixation is required for multilevel anterior corpectomy performed at three or more vertebral levels in order to ensure adequate construct stabilization. Traction may be used if the patient has a severe kyphotic deformity in the cervical spine or if subluxation is present.

The anterolateral approach to the subaxial cervical spine represents a relatively atraumatic spinal dissection with a generous exposure allowing for access to a wide range of spinal pathologies. An intraoperative tracheostomy, PEG, or nasogastric (NG) tube may be placed, as postoperative edema can compress the airway and esophagus. Additional care should be given for patients who previously received radiation treatments because scarring and tissue deterioration can significantly increase the risk of complications. Esophageal erosion from anterior plate hardware is a rare but serious complication with a reported incidence of 1.49%, and the patient should be monitored long term for any symptoms of instrumentation failure.[20]

Thoracic Spine

Metastatic tumors in the thoracic region represent 70% of metastatic disease in the spine.[3] One of the primary anatomic advantages for surgical resection of tumors in the thoracic region is that, if necessary, nerve roots can be easily ligated without severe functional deficit. In addition, the thoracic spine is more stable than other spinal regions because it is mechanically reinforced by the ribs and sternum.

Anterior Neck Dissection and Sternotomy

First described by Rosen et al,[21] this approach provides the most direct access to the cervicothoracic junction (as high as C4) and to the superior aspect of the T3 vertebral body. The patient is positioned supine with towels under the scapula to extend the neck slightly. A T-shaped incision is made 1 cm above the clavicle with a vertically oriented medial incision over the sternum (**Fig. 5.2b**). Once exposure is established, a rectangular block of sternum is resected along with about one third of the clavicle on the operative side. Although entry from the left is preferred due to the risk of injury to the right recurrent laryngeal nerve, the approach should also be dictated by the side with the greatest extravertebral tumor extension. Instrumentation following low cervical/high thoracic vertebrectomy that does not extend across the cervicothoracic transition zone

will often lead to a higher incidence of adjacent level degeneration due to added mechanical stress. As a result, this approach facilitates good visualization and proper screw and plate placement across the cervicothoracic junction.

The presence of an anterolateral soft tissue mass is viewed as a contraindication for such an approach due to the already limited operative space available. Considering the relatively small operative field and the anatomic complexity of the upper thoracic cavity, this approach presents a challenge to most spinal surgeons. Patients must be made aware of the possibility of an intraoperative tracheostomy and gastrostomy, pulmonary injury, the risks of recurrent laryngeal nerve palsy, and the potential for damage to the great vessels.[22]

Case Illustration

A 39-year-old woman presented with breast cancer with diffuse skeletal and spinal metastases despite chemotherapy (**Fig. 5.3a**). The lytic nature of the lesions at C6 and C7 resulted in vertebra plana, with complete loss of the vertebral body height. She developed paraplegia, and underwent radiation therapy and external immobilization and recovered the ability to ambulate with some assistance. A staged surgical procedure was offered. The patient underwent preoperative reduction with 35 pounds of traction with gradual correction of her deformity. The first stage of the surgery included a left anterior cervical approach and median sternotomy to gain access to the left cervicothoracic junction. The anterior corpectomy was performed through an aortocaval window above the pulmonary artery and below the innominate vein. The vertebral bodies of C6-T1 were removed using a high-speed diamond bur. Decompression of the C6-T1 nerve roots was also performed. An anterior cage and plate were placed extending from C5 to T2. Four days later, a C5-T1 bilateral total laminectomy and a C2-T8 posterior fixation completed the second stage of the procedure (**Fig. 5.3b**). Her clinical course was complicated by facial edema, bilateral pleural effusions, and hospital-acquired pneumonia. She was discharged to rehabilitation and survived 3½ years after surgery.

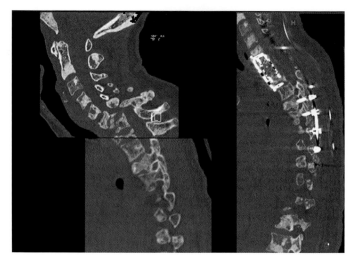

a   b

Fig. 5.3a,b Metastatic lesion at the cervicothoracic junction. **(a)** Composite cervical and thoracic preoperative computed tomography (CT) scan from a patient with metastatic breast cancer in the cervicothoracic junction demonstrating vertebra plana of C6-C7 with focal kyphosis and grade 4 anterolisthesis. Intraoperatively, the vertebral bodies of C6-T1 were removed using a high-speed diamond bur. **(b)** An anterior cage and plate were placed extending from C5-T2. Four days later, C5-T1 bilateral laminectomy and C2-T8 posterior fixation completed the second stage of the procedure.

The "Trapdoor" Approach

The "trapdoor" exposure can be performed bilaterally and differs from the above transsternal approach by providing extended visualization of the T3-T4 region. Anatomically, the T3-T4 region rests behind the great vessels and heart, which makes it inaccessible from the approaches described above. As a result, the trapdoor approach provides a more lateral exposure by further opening the thoracic cavity to enable the mobilization of anterior elements. The patient is positioned supine similarly to the sternotomy approach. The initial incision is made along the medial border of the sternocleidomastoid muscle to the sternal notch and is then extended ventrally over the fourth interspace (**Fig. 5.2c**). Although this approach is similar to the transsternal approach in that the neck is fully dissected, it differs in that there is no need for the clavicle to be transected. Significant retraction is placed on the sternal retractor so as to open the "trapdoor" and provide access to the thoracic cavity. Dual lobe intubation is required to allow the ipsilateral lung to be deflated, exposing the C4-T4 vertebral bodies for cage placement if necessary (**Fig. 5.4a**).

Unlike other anterior approaches, the trapdoor exposure preserves the clavicle and sternoclavicular junction. Due to the manipulation of the great vessels and violation of the thoracic cavity, great attention should be given postoperatively to monitoring the patient for symptoms of hemopericardium, particularly following previous irradiation. Symptoms include cardiac tamponade, shortness of breath, and chest pain. Treatment consists of the insertion of a needle into the pericardial window for pericardial drainage. Although the increased risk of morbidity and the lengthy postoperative care are potential contraindications for the treatment of metastases, this approach provides the best anterior visualization of the T3-T4 vertebral bodies. Alternatively, an anterolateral approach can be performed to gain access to the same spinal region and is preferred by some surgeons.[23]

Thoracotomy (Transthoracic Approach)

By providing a wide anterior surgical field, the thoracotomy or transthoracic approach provides

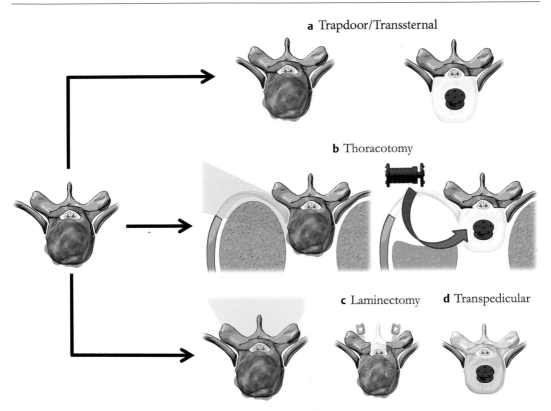

Fig. 5.4a–d Methods for approaching the thoracic spine. **(a)** Anterior access to the upper thoracic spine via the trapdoor or transsternal approach. **(b)** Thoracotomy (transthoracic) approach for anterior decompression followed by anterior cage and plate fixation. **(c)** Posterior decompression via laminectomy followed by instrumentation. **(d)** Posterior vertebrectomy using the transpedicular approach with subsequent cage placement.

access to the ipsilateral pedicle, the thoracic vertebral bodies, the nerve roots, and the spinal canal. Compared with the posterior approach, the transthoracic approach affords a wider view and permits maximal decompression while minimizing manipulation of the spinal cord for access to ventral pathology.

The patient is placed in a lateral decubitus position with the arm extended outward in order to elevate the scapula off the chest wall. The rhomboids and trapezius muscles are then incised on the lower edge of the scapula enabling visualization of the underlying ribs. This approach can be divided into two techniques based on the anatomic considerations of the thoracic spine, namely high (T5-T7) and low thoracotomy (T7-T10). For a high thoracotomy, the scapula must be mobilized. As with other approaches, the operative side should be chosen based on the tumor pathology; however, the left side is anatomically preferable because the spleen is easier to retract than the liver and the aorta easier to repair than the vena cava. In patients who have undergone previous chest surgery, it is preferable to choose the naïve side in order to avoid pleural adhesions that may increase the risk of postoperative pneumo- and hemothorax.

For lesions involving T5-T6, the rib corresponding to the tumor level is removed. Given the curvature of the ribs, at the T7-T8 levels, the rib one level above the tumor is removed. Likewise for the T9-T10 levels, the rib that is two levels above the tumor is removed to provide adequate visualization of the vertebral body.[23] Once the rib is resected, the parietal pleura is exposed and the ribs are spread using a self-retaining retractor. Intubation with a dual-lumen endotracheal tube enables complete or partial deflation of a single lung. The pleural space provides a plane of dissection and the surgeon can gently retract the lung and parietal pleura away from the surgical field. This will provide exposure of the affected vertebral body, which may be resected piecemeal or en bloc with the use of a Tomita saw. A cage may then be placed if reconstruction is necessary (**Fig. 5.4b**). Air leaks may be assessed by filling the thoracic cavity with saline and examining for air bubbles. Upon completion of the surgery, two chests tubes may be placed: the inferior chest tube is placed at the posterior corner of the diaphragm to collect blood, and the other tube is placed at the apex of the lung to allow trapped air to escape.

Pulmonary compromise resulting from lung metastases is a relative contraindication to thoracotomy. Complications include pneumonia, airway obstruction, atelectasis, pneumothorax, pleural effusion, and hemothorax. The risk of these complications is substantially increased in elderly patients, and careful assessment of preoperative lung function is necessary before surgery.

Transpedicular Approach

The transpedicular approach utilizes posterior exposure to access anterior pathology. This can reduce the size of the incision and enable circumferential decompression and cage placement when bilateral transpedicular approaches are used. The patient is place prone and a midline incision is made extending up to two levels above and below the level of the tumor. The length of the incision is dictated by the planned instrumentation. Laminectomies are performed to provide posterior decompression of the cord (**Fig. 5.4c**). The facet joints, the proximal transverse processes, and the pedicles are subsequently removed, providing access to the rostral and caudal intervertebral disk. Once the plane between the posterior longitudinal ligament (PLL) and the dura is identified, the PLL in incised at the disk space above and below the origin of disease. The tumor and vertebral body are then resected piecewise until there is ade-

quate space for expandable cage and allograft insertion (**Fig. 5.4d**). It is important to completely remove any cartilaginous tissue from both end plates to ensure proper cage fixation. Posterior fixation with pedicle screws and fitted rods is then performed to support the anterior construct and prevent forward translation of the superior adjacent vertebral body.

The separation of the PLL from the dura via the posterior approach should be performed with extreme caution. Unintended durotomy may result if the tumor is calcified or if adjacent disk herniations are calcified, compromising the plane between the PLL and dura. If a CSF leak results and a CSF fistula or pseudomeningocele forms, a lumbar drain can be placed to divert CSF flow. In the case of an epidural hematoma from spinal cord manipulation, immediate evacuation should be performed. In addition, the placement of the interbody cage can often be challenging due to the restricted operative window available.

Thoracoabdominal Approach

This approach combines a low posterolateral thoracotomy with the retroperitoneal approach for visualization of the thoracolumbar region (T11-L1). A left-sided approach is preferred. The patient is placed in a lateral decubitus position and an incision is made over the 10th rib, extending from the paraspinous muscles anteriorly to the costal cartilage (**Fig. 5.5a,b**). Because the diaphragm attaches to the 11th and 12th ribs, if resection of these ribs is warranted, the diaphragm is incised circumferentially leaving a 2-inch cuff of tissue to facilitate closure. The ipsilateral lung is deflated using a dual-lumen endotracheal tube and is retracted, enabling access to the retroperitoneal cavity, which can be navigated with blunt dissection to the diaphragmatic crus (**Fig. 5.5c**). Incision of the proximal attachment of the ipsilateral psoas can provide additional exposure of the vertebral body. Although breach of the peritoneal cavity is preferably avoided, if it occurs, the tear should be either closed or extended so as to prevent the strangulation of the bowel via hiatal hernia formation. In addition to the risks

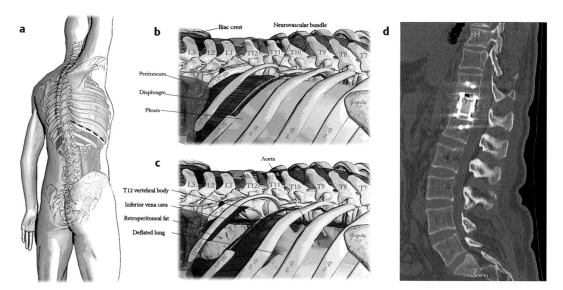

Fig. 5.5a–d Thoracoabdominal approach for access to T12. **(a)** The patient's arm is extended and an incision is made over the 10th rib. **(b)** Once exposure of the diaphragm is granted, the ipsilateral lung is deflated. **(c)** Retroperitoneal fat, which lies behind the diaphragm, is retracted along with peritoneum providing access to the T12 vertebral body (*bright yellow*). **(d)** Sagittal CT scan demonstrating cage and place placement following T12 vertebral body resection in a patient with metastatic colon carcinoma.

posed to the thoracotomy approach, the thoracoabdominal approach also risks injury to the spleen, kidney and ureters.

Case Illustration

A 47-year-old man presented with intractable back pain requiring daily treatment with a high-dose fentanyl patch. The patient had a past medical history of metastatic colon carcinoma and had received chemotherapy and radiation to a lesion at T12. He had a mass in the left lung, suspicious for a pulmonary metastasis. Surgery was offered when imaging demonstrated a progressive kyphosis at the T12 level and a wedge deformity of the T12 vertebral body. Intraoperative imaging was used to identify the 10th rib, and an overlying incision was made. The rib was excised and the chest cavity was entered. The diaphragm was detached from the chest wall, a rectangular incision was made in the parietal pleura, and the iliopsoas was mobilized. T11-12 and T12-L1 diskectomies were performed, followed by piecemeal resection of the T12 vertebral body until the PLL was visibly decompressed. The cage was then placed between T11 and L1 to restore anatomic alignment (**Fig 5.5d**). The cage was packed with allograft bone from the 10th rib and a plate was placed extending from T11 to L1. A single chest tube was placed and the diaphragm was closed using 1-0 Prolene. Postoperatively, the patient complained of decreased lung capacity and feeling winded, and he died 3 months after surgery.

■ Lumbar Spine

Approximately one in every five spine tumor cases occurs in the lumbar region.[3] The lumbar spine is unique in that, inferior to the conus medullaris, the cord becomes the branched cauda equina. In patients with metastases to the lumbar spine, preexisting lumbar degenerative scoliosis and disk disease may complicate the surgical approach and planning. In patients with a greater than 30-degree Cobb angle, with lateral translation of the vertebral bodies, or severe spondylolisthesis, simple decompression alone may worsen their degenerative lumbar spine disease. Clinical assessment and surgical planning should take comorbid pathology into account. Flexion and extension radiographs are advised if spondylolisthesis is suspected.

Posterior Approach (Laminectomy)

A posterior approach to the lumbar spine can be sufficient for palliative care of anterior pathologies. Posterior decompression via laminectomy or foraminotomy with posterior fixation is one of the best known surgical techniques with a very low rate of postoperative complications. However, there is growing evidence that suggests that laminectomy alone for decompression is no more effective than radiation in treating neurologic pain.[24]

Retroperitoneal Approach

The retroperitoneal approach provides anterior access to the lumbar spine in tumor cases to enable effective resection and to restore anterior column stability. The patient is placed in a semilateral (45-degree) decubitus position and the table is arched so as to widen the space between the hip and ribs. An oblique flank incision is made between the 12th rib and the iliac crest centered at the tumor level. The internal oblique and the transversus abdominis muscle layers are divided in line with the skin incision, exposing retroperitoneal fat, which is then retracted anteriorly along with peritoneum. Once the vertebral level is confirmed, ligation of the segmental vessels enables mobilization of the aorta to facilitate exposure of the anterior part of the vertebral body. A corpectomy can then be performed using a diamond bur for circumferential decompression of the spinal cord. Incomplete resection of the contralateral pedicle can be avoided by further tilting the patient so as to enhance visualization. Once the anterior vertebral body and adjacent vertebral disks are removed, the PLL should be carefully dissected away from the cord. This facilitates exposure of

both nerve roots and reduces the risk of radicular pain caused by root compression.

Care should be taken to avoid entering either the perirenal fat or the retropsoas space—two regions that are commonly incurred instead of the plane in front of the quadratus lumborum and psoas muscles.[23] Both the ureter and genitofemoral nerve should be protected from excessive retraction. Unlike the thoracic spine, anterior approaches to the lumbar spine pose an additional challenge because the nerve roots should be preserved whenever possible. For approaches involving the lower lumbar spine, it should be taken into consideration that the aorta bifurcates into the common iliac vessels at L4. Mobilization of the great vessels by a vascular access surgeon may be required for exposure of L3-L4.

■ Sacral Approaches

Although rare, malignant tumors of the sacral spine present a complex array of challenges. Due to the delayed onset of symptoms, patients often present with large tumors with some degree of adjacent structure invasion at the time of their diagnosis. If resection constitutes greater than 50% of the sacroiliac (SI) joint, reconstruction with a transiliac bar, femoral graft, iliac, and pedicle screws is necessary.[25]

Sacrectomy has proven effective in treating a number of sacral tumors; however, the literature describing sacral tumor resection includes a majority of patients with primary spinal tumors. The degree of sacrectomy (low, middle, high, or total) is dependent on a number of factors including the tumor pathology, the nerve roots involved, and subsequent goals of surgery. Knowledge of sacral vascular anatomy is crucial for sacrectomy approaches. The aorta bifurcates to form the common iliac arteries at the level of the L3-4 disk, and the common iliac arteries become the internal and external iliacs at the lumbosacral articulation. Bilaterally, the common iliacs are transversed by the ureter. The common iliacs give off the medial and lateral sacral arteries, which commonly supply presacral tumors. The superior and inferior gluteal arteries also traverse the sacrum. Significant bleeding can result from injury to these arteries.

Because the majority of tumors occur anteriorly, sacrectomies are typically performed in a two-stage, anterior then posterior, fashion. The principal aims of the anterior approach are to expose the anterior aspects of the tumor, dissect adhesions to the bowel and abdominal viscera, and ligate the main vessels.[26] The patient is placed in a supine position and a midline incision is made extending from the umbilicus to the symphysis pubis to expose the anterior lumbosacral region. The ureters and iliac vessels are carefully dissected and preserved. A vascular access surgeon may assist in mobilization of the great vessels. If necessary, a colostomy can be performed at this stage of the operation to protect the bowel from later radiation or if the bowel is invaded by the tumor.

The periosteum is then identified and dissected. Midline osteotomies may be scored into the bone following exposure. The lumbar trunk and lumbosacral plexus are then identified and preserved along the lateral aspect of the sacral ala. Lateral to the plexus, the sacroiliac joint can be identified, and bilateral sacroiliac osteotomies are performed if total sacrectomy is merited. The L5-S1 disk and annulus are then incised. A Silastic sheath may be placed posterior to the vascular structures and the rectum to prevent adhesions. If a large sacral defect is planned, a myocutaneous flap, such as a ventral rectus abdominis myocutaneous (VRAM) flap is then prepared, fed by the inferior epigastric vessels.

High-volume blood loss may complicate the anterior procedure, and, if necessary, the posterior approach may be performed several days after the first operation. For this approach, the patient is placed prone and a midline incision is made extending from L2 inferiorly past the coccyx. A laminectomy is performed at L5 and S1 to expose the cauda equina and nerve roots. Lateral sacroiliac osteotomies are performed, meeting the anterior osteotomies. Although there is little reported in the literature, several groups have reported success using the modified Galveston L-rod technique for spinopelvic reconstruction.[27] Autograft and demineralized bone are placed in the defect to promote fusion, and the rectus abdominis flap is used to reconstruct the defect. Gluteal flaps are also mobilized medially to serve as additional protection. The single-stage posterior approach has also been successfully used for sacrectomy, reducing the wound size and reducing the potential risk for vascular complications.[28] Further, if the tumor does not violate more than 50% of the SI joint, the caudal extent of the sacrum may be removed without any spinopelvic reconstruction.

There are a number of possible complications associated with sacrectomy. Impairment of the sacral nerve roots often results in urologic, anorectal, and sexual function issues. In one study, Todd et al[29] reported that the preservation of at least one S3 nerve root preserves satisfactory bowel and bladder function in most patients. Preservation of bilateral S1 is required for normal ambulation. In addition, reconstruction of the spinopelvis can result in loss of ambulation and vertical and rotation instability of the lower spine. There is also an increased risk of deep wound infections and major wound dehiscence.

■ Role of Minimally Invasive Surgery

Minimally invasive surgery (MIS) has emerged as an approach for patients with metastatic spine disease to reduce blood loss, operative time, and complication rates, although class I evidence is lacking.[30] Several common MIS approaches such as endoscopy, thoracoscopy, and laparoscopy can provide effective access for vertebroplasty, corpectomy, and percutaneous screw placement throughout the spine. MIS has great potential for reducing postoperative pain and complications such as wound dehiscence.[21,30] Specifically, for patients with spinal metastases who are eligible for adjuvant therapy, MIS techniques result in smaller wounds and may decrease wound healing time. This can decrease the time from surgery to adminis-tration of chemotherapy or radiation therapy. However, there is a steep learning curve with these approaches, and the exposure can be lim-ited compared with that of open techniques. Furthermore, few reports have demonstrated success using MIS to provide circumferential spinal cord decompression and stabilization for the treatment of tumors. As a result, MIS may be a useful technique in a carefully selected population of patients.

■ Chapter Summary

To a large extent, treatment for patients with metastatic cancer often remains palliative due to the presence of lesions at multiple foci. When considering surgical intervention, there are four primary objectives: reduction of intractable pain; preservation/improvement of neurologic function; correction of mechanical instability; and oncological control. In general, approaches to the spine can be divided into three catego-ries: anterior, posterior, or combined. Although metastatic tumors primarily originate anteriorly, direct access to the anterior spine presents a number of operative challenges including lim-ited access, increased risk of comorbidity, and extended hospital recovery time. In the past, the workhorse technique of most metastatic lesions was posterior decompression via lami-nectomy and instrumented fixation. However, several posterior/posterolateral approaches have been developed to address the issue of circum-ferential decompression of the spinal cord. As nonsurgical treatments continue to improve, patients will continue to demonstrate longer median survival times that will facilitate the use of en bloc resection for long-term pain re-lief. Although several of the techniques men-tioned are considered technically demanding,

surgical outcomes are greatly dependent on the experience of the surgical team. Knowledge of spinal anatomy and how to properly address intraoperative complications is critical for pa-tient success.

Pearls

- Prior to any intervention for spinal metastatic dis-ease, review the patient's anatomy to determine the role of comorbid degenerative pathology.
- For anterior approaches to the cervical spine, con-sider preoperative tracheostomy and PEG or NG tube placement to provide ventilation and nutri-tion in the event of severe perioperative airway edema.
- A misplaced lateral mass screw in a single verte-bral artery will tamponade the damaged vessel until endovascular repair is available.
- Intubation with a dual-lumen endotracheal tube allows deflation of a single lung for thoracic tumor approaches.
- In the thoracic spine, sacrifice of nerve roots re-sults in minimal patient morbidity and improved exposure.
- For thoracolumbar approaches, the aorta is more difficult to injure and easier to repair than the vena cava; thus, a left-sided approach is preferred.
- Resection of greater than 50% of the SI joint re-quires its reconstruction with femoral or fibular strut allograft with transiliac rods and iliac screws.

Pitfalls

- Esophageal perforation is a rare, late complica-tion following anterior cervical plating.
- Never place a screw in the contralateral lateral mass following injury to the vertebral artery.
- Hemo- and pneumothorax are common compli-cations following thoracotomy approaches, and postoperative chest tube placement helps to de-crease these risks.
- Cardiac tamponade from hemopericardium is a rare but life-threatening complication following sternal approaches and can be temporarily man-aged with a pericardial window for drainage of blood.

References

Five Must-Read References

1. Marchesi DG, Boos N, Aebi M. Surgical treatment of tumors of the cervical spine and first two thoracic vertebrae. J Spinal Disord 1993;6:489–496
2. Galasko CS. Skeletal metastases. Clin Orthop Relat Res 1986;210:18–30
3. Perrin RG, McBroom RJ. Anterior versus posterior decompression for symptomatic spinal metastasis. Can J Neurol Sci 1987;14:75–80
4. Cavaliere R, Schiff D. Epidural spinal cord compression. Curr Treat Options Neurol 2004;6:285–295
5. Quraishi NA, Purushothamdas S, Manoharan SR, Arealis G, Lenthall R, Grevitt MP. Outcome of embolised vascular metastatic renal cell tumours causing spinal cord compression. Eur Spine J 2013;22(Suppl 1):S27–S32
6. Sciubba DM, Petteys RJ, Dekutoski MB, et al. Diagnosis and management of metastatic spine disease. A review. J Neurosurg Spine 2010;13:94–108
7. Patchell RA, Tibbs PA, Regine WF, et al. Direct decompressive surgical resection in the treatment of spinal cord compression caused by metastatic cancer: a randomised trial. Lancet 2005;366:643–648
8. Tokuhashi Y, Matsuzaki H, Toriyama S, Kawano H, Ohsaka S. Scoring system for the preoperative evaluation of metastatic spine tumor prognosis. Spine 1990;15:1110–1113
9. Tomita K, Kawahara N, Kobayashi T, Yoshida A, Murakami H, Akamaru T. Surgical strategy for spinal metastases. Spine 2001;26:298–306
10. Fisher CG, DiPaola CP, Ryken TC, et al. A novel classification system for spinal instability in neoplastic disease: an evidence-based approach and expert consensus from the Spine Oncology Study Group. Spine 2010;35:E1221–E1229
11. Cloyd JM, Acosta FL Jr, Polley MY, Ames CP. En bloc resection for primary and metastatic tumors of the spine: a systematic review of the literature. Neurosurgery 2010;67:435–444, discussion 444–445
12. Fehlings MG, David KS, Vialle L, Vialle E, Setzer M, Vrionis FD. Decision making in the surgical treatment of cervical spine metastases. Spine 2009;34(22, Suppl):S108–S117
13. Molina CA, Gokaslan ZL, Sciubba DM. Diagnosis and management of metastatic cervical spine tumors. Orthop Clin North Am 2012;43:75–87, viii–ix viii–ix
14. Wright NM, Lauryssen C; American Association of Neurological Surgeons/Congress of Neurological Surgeons. Vertebral artery injury in C1-2 transarticular screw fixation: results of a survey of the AANS/CNS section on disorders of the spine and peripheral nerves. J Neurosurg 1998;88:634–640
15. Hsu W, Wolinsky JP, Gokaslan ZL, Sciubba DM. Transoral approaches to the cervical spine. Neurosurgery 2010;66(3, Suppl):119–125
16. Hannallah D, Lee J, Khan M, Donaldson WF, Kang JD. Cerebrospinal fluid leaks following cervical spine surgery. J Bone Joint Surg Am 2008;90:1101–1105
17. Bhatia R, Desouza RM, Bull J, Casey AT. Rigid occipitocervical fixation: indications, outcomes, and complications in the modern era. J Neurosurg Spine 2013; 18:333–339
18. Menezes AH. Surgical approaches: postoperative care and complications "transoral-transpalatopharyngeal approach to the craniocervical junction". Childs Nerv Syst 2008;24:1187–1193
19. Smith GW, Robinson RA. The treatment of certain cervical-spine disorders by anterior removal of the intervertebral disc and interbody fusion. J Bone Joint Surg Am 1958;40-A:607–624
20. Gaudinez RF, English GM, Gebhard JS, Brugman JL, Donaldson DH, Brown CW. Esophageal perforations after anterior cervical surgery. J Spinal Disord 2000; 13:77–84
21. Rosen DS, O'Toole JE, Eichholz KM, et al. Minimally invasive lumbar spinal decompression in the elderly: outcomes of 50 patients aged 75 years and older. Neurosurgery 2007;60:503–509, discussion 509–510
22. Resnick DK. Anterior cervicothoracic junction corpectomy and plate fixation without sternotomy. Neurosurg Focus 2002;12:E7
23. Fourney DR, Gokaslan ZL. Anterior approaches for thoracolumbar metastatic spine tumors. Neurosurg Clin N Am 2004;15:443–451
24. Klimo P Jr, Dailey AT, Fessler RG. Posterior surgical approaches and outcomes in metastatic spine-disease. Neurosurg Clin N Am 2004;15:425–435
25. Gunterberg B, Romanus B, Stener B. Pelvic strength after major amputation of the sacrum. An exerimental study. Acta Orthop Scand 1976;47:635–642
26. Fourney D, Gokaslan Z. Surgical approaches for the resection of sacral tumors. In: Dickman C, Fehlings M, Gokaslan Z, eds. Spinal Cord and Spinal Column Tumors: Principles and Practice. New York: Thieme Medical, 2006:632–648
27. Gokaslan ZL, Romsdahl MM, Kroll SS, et al. Total sacrectomy and Galveston L-rod reconstruction for malignant neoplasms. Technical note. J Neurosurg 1997; 87:781–787
28. Clarke MJ, Dasenbrock H, Bydon A, et al. Posterioronly approach for en bloc sacrectomy: clinical outcomes in 36 consecutive patients. Neurosurgery 2012;71:357–364, discussion 364

29. Todd LT Jr, Yaszemski MJ, Currier BL, Fuchs B, Kim CW, Sim FH. Bowel and bladder function after major sacral resection. Clin Orthop Relat Res 2002;397: 36–39

30. Molina CA, Gokaslan ZL, Sciubba DM. A systematic review of the current role of minimally invasive spine surgery in the management of metastatic spine disease. Int J Surg Oncol 2011;2011:598148

6

Spinal Reconstruction and Fixation/Fusion

Rajiv Saigal and Dean Chou

■ Introduction

Surgery for metastatic spinal tumors was once a controversial topic, due to meager outcomes from decompressive laminectomy and unclear benefits compared to radiation alone.[1–3] However, as surgical practice advanced to include metastatic tumor resection and spinal fixation/stabilization,[4] neurologic outcome and pain results began to improve.[1] The landmark 2005 Patchell et al[5] study definitively changed management, establishing that circumferential surgical decompression plus adjuvant radiation is a favorable therapeutic strategy for patients with neurologic deficit from epidural spinal cord compression and an expected survival of at least 3 months.

Strategies for spinal reconstruction and fixation have only grown in importance since, with around 25,000 new cases of metastatic epidural spinal cord compression yearly in the United States.[6] After pulmonary and hepatic sites, the skeletal system is the next most common site of metastasis, and the spinal column is the most common skeletal site.[6] When the pathological vertebral body is removed, the spinal column must be reconstructed in order to provide structural support. Reconstruction after resection of metastasis can generally be undertaken from an anterior, posterior, or combined approach. Techniques for vertebral body reconstruction vary widely, from the early use of polymethylmethacrylate with Steinmann

pins[7] or chest tubes[8] to the more modern use of expandable titanium cages.[9] Here we discuss clinical issues and preoperative planning, and summarize the key points and supporting data for each of these methods.

■ Preoperative Planning

Preoperative planning for spinal reconstruction cases is vital to ensure operative success. Planning includes acquiring adequate imaging, deciding whether to use an approach surgeon and whether to complete the procedure as a single stage or in multiple stages, considering preoperative tumor embolization, and scheduling the required equipment, including implanted hardware systems and neuromonitoring.

Imaging Modalities

Magnetic resonance imaging (MRI), computed tomography (CT), and plain film X-rays provide unique, complementary information in preparation for metastasis removal with spine reconstruction. As part of cancer staging, positron emission tomography (PET) or nuclear scintigraphy scans may often provide the first diagnosis of metastatic spinal cord compression, but generally they do not provide adequate resolution for preoperative planning.[6] A contrast MRI scan helps to delineate the tumor boundaries and the degree of epidural spinal cord compression. MRI can clarify whether a metastatic tumor is confined to the vertebral body or extends to the posterior elements. CT best defines the bony anatomy; in addition to assessing the pathological bone invaded by tumor, the surgeon can assess bone quality at adjacent segments. Preoperative measurement of pedicle size and anatomy enables optimization of pedicle screw diameter, length, and trajectory. CT myelogram may be performed in patients with contraindications to MRI, such as implanted pacemakers or deep brain stimulators, but it carries the downside of being an invasive procedure with its own intrinsic risks. Standing or sitting spine X-rays demonstrate the effects of load-bearing, information unavailable from the standard supine spine MRI or CT scan. Sagittal and coronal balance should also be measured on weight-bearing X-rays (if possible), not on supine MRIs or CTs, in order to establish a preoperative baseline.

Presurgical planning also involves deciding what type of intraoperative imaging to order. Anteroposterior (AP) and lateral C-arm fluoroscopy is used for localization in most cases. Intraoperative CT (when available) and navigation can be used for real-time image-guided implant placement or for ensuring proper placement of implants.

The Surgical Team

It is sometimes beneficial to utilize an approach surgeon an approach surgeon who has expertise in anterior or lateral approaches. If anterior access to the upper cervical spine (C1-2) is required, an otolaryngologist–head and neck surgeon may be required for transoral approaches with or without mandible splitting. A thoracic surgeon is required for sternotomy for anterior access to the thoracic spine and may be beneficial for lateral thoracic approaches.[10] A general or vascular surgeon may provide anterior retroperitoneal access to the lumbosacral spine. Even for spine surgeons who are trained in anterior and lateral approaches, it may be advantageous to arrange the services of an approach surgeon who has experience dealing with unexpected occurrences and maximizing patient safety. Region-specific approaches are discussed in greater detail in Chapter 5.

Staging

For cases that involve expected long operative time or multiple anatomic approaches, some surgeons would consider staging in order to facilitate patient tolerance and to reduce surgeon fatigue. However, there is growing evidence to suggest that performing anterior and posterior fusions on separate days is not beneficial. A single-stage procedure may entail decreased overall operative time, lower blood loss, better deformity correction, and shorter hospital stay.[11–13] In a recent study of the Nationwide Inpatient Sample, a 28% complication rate was observed with staged anterior-posterior surgeries, a significant increase over the 22% rate for same-day surgeries.[12] With staging, there were increased rates of venous thrombosis and acute respiratory distress syndrome with no mortality benefit.

Angiography and Embolization

Thoughtful consideration should be given to the option of preoperative angiogram with embolization in highly vascular lesions. A neurointerventional radiologist or endovascular neurosurgeon should be consulted for lesions deemed amenable to angiography or embolization. Angiography alone may be valuable to identify the segmental level and side of the artery of Adamkiewicz, especially when considering anterior or lateral approaches between T9 and L2.[14,15] However, magnetic resonance (MR) or CT angiography should be considered as less invasive methods to obtain the same anatomic information. For certain hypervascular tumors, such as renal cell carcinoma, thyroid carcinoma, hepatocellular carcinoma, or hemangiopericytoma, preoperative embolization may minimize blood loss, enhancing safety and reducing operative time. However, embolization itself carries the risk of neurologic compromise. In one series, three of 12 patients (25%) suffered neurologic deficits after preoperative embolization.[8] Therefore, risks and benefits must be carefully weighed prior to proceeding.

Neuromonitoring

Intraoperative neuromonitoring is commonly used for spine reconstruction with implants, although there is a paucity of data showing effect on neurologic outcomes. For cases with partial or no preoperative motor or sensory deficit, motor evoked potentials (MEPs) and somatosensory evoked potentials (SSEPs) provide important feedback to the surgeon about whether any surgical manipulations nerve roots, albeit with the inherent risk of false negatives. An exception would be the case of complete spinal cord injury from metastatic spinal cord compression. Even in such cases, some clinicians would consider using preoperative MEPs and SSEPs to confirm a suspected complete spinal cord injury based on neurologic exam. For unstable spine lesions, preoperative supine MEPs and SSEPs are imperative to establish whether patient positioning causes any departure from baseline before the surgery commences. Additionally, direct stimulation of implanted screws intraoperatively may alert the surgeon to the presence of an unexpected breach from the intended trajectory.

■ Approaches

Anterior Approach

Anterior approaches have long been used for resection of vertebral body metastasis with reconstruction of the anterior column. An established technique in the thoracic spine entails anterior vertebrectomy, decompression, and reconstruction. The main benefits of an anterior approach are direct access to the diseased segment(s), improved wound healing, biomechanical strength from weight-bearing column reconstruction, and fixation of fewer segments.[8] There are various options for vertebral body reconstruction supplemented with locking plate and screws.

The anterior approach requires careful consideration of anatomic restraints and generally requires assistance of an approach surgeon. At T1-2, a combined anterior neck dissection and sternotomy is favored.[8] At T3-4, an anterior neck dissection with partial sternotomy and anterolateral thoracotomy enables "trapdoor" entry to the chest cavity.[8] T5-10 is less favorable for a pure anterior approach due to anatomic location of the heart, aortic arch, and great vessels; a right-sided thoracotomy is favored.[6] At T11-L1, an anterior thoracotomy or anterior retroperitoneal approach may be necessary. Retroperitoneal approaches are generally used in the lumbar spine.[16]

Prior to commencing the vertebrectomy, segmental vessels should be identified, ligated, and transected. The intervertebral disks rostral and caudal to the pathological segments(s) should be removed with an annulotomy knife, rongeurs, and curettes. After removing cartilaginous layers, care should be taken to minimize the removal of subchondral cortical bone.[9] Removal of end-plate bone increases the risk of graft subsidence. Vertebrectomy and removal of metastatic tissue then follows. The use of Leksell rongeurs at the outset enables the removal of larger pieces of diseased tissue and relative structural preservation in specimens sent to the pathology lab for diagnosis. A high-speed drill with a round or matchstick drill bit is necessary to remove posterior vertebral body tissue, particularly when nearing the posterior longitudinal ligament. An ultrasonic aspirator can be used to assist with tumor removal. The posterior longitudinal ligament is often opened to facilitate visualization of the underlying spinal cord dura and exiting nerve roots. A thorough decompression can only be ensured with direct visualization.

Options for anterior column reconstruction include auto- or allograft bone, static and expandable cages, polyetheretherketone (PEEK) cages, and polymethylmethacrylate (PMMA) augmented with Steinmann pins. Prior to the widespread availability of mesh cages, PMMA was often used to fill in the vertebrectomy defect, historically combined with either a Steinmann pin or a chest tube as a scaffold. To accomplish the latter, a cylindrical defect was drilled into the superior and inferior vertebrae. A chest tube was cut to size and filled with PMMA.[8] In an exothermic polymerization process, PMMA can heat surrounding tissues, so irrigation with lukewarm saline is beneficial.[8] PMMA provides large surface area coverage of the end plate to minimize subsidence and is extremely stable and strong in compression.

A more modern method of anterior column reconstruction entails the use of an expandable titanium cage.[9] Expandable cages are increasingly employed due to their facility of use, restoration of vertebral height, and improvement in sagittal alignment and mechanical strength. Correction of sagittal alignment is a major advantage over methylmethacrylate, but higher cost is a disadvantage.

After anterior column reconstruction, supporting instrumentation is implanted. An anterior locking plate with screws prevents distraction and stabilizes implants.[8] In patients with poor bone quality or significant kyphosis, anterior fixation alone does not restore stability comparable to healthy segments in the thoracolumbar spine,[17] and additional posterior supplementation should be considered in patients with extended life expectancy. When operating in the thoracic cavity, chest tubes are left in place during the early postoperative period.

Although providing direct access, anterior thoracotomy approaches carry the highest complication rate: 39% (including 3.5% reoperation rate and 1.5% mortality); lateral extracavitary and costotransversectomy approaches carry lower morbidity rates of 17% and 15%, respectively.[18] Despite the high complication rate, 76% of patients with neurologic compromise at presentation improved in some series.[8]

Posterior-Only Approaches

Costotransversectomy, transpedicular, and extracavitary approaches are viable options for posterior-only reconstruction in the lumbar[19] and thoracic[20] spine. They offer the benefit of anterior column reconstruction and posterior supplementation from a single approach. In addition, comorbidities or anatomic tumor burdens may preclude an anterior thoracic or abdominal approach and thus require a posterior-only approach. The three approaches differ in the degree of rib removal involved. The standard extracavitary approach requires removal of a substantial amount of rib with pleural dissection in order to access the spine. Costotransversectomies involve removal of the rib head in approaching the spine. Transpedicular corpectomies are performed entirely through the pedicle and do not require removal of the rib head nor pleural dissection. More commonly today these three approaches have been combined into one posterolateral approach; essentially whatever bone is needed to be removed to accomplish the surgical goals of decompression and reconstruction is removed. For placement of methylmethacrylate supplemented with Steinmann pins, a thin rim of cortical bone if often left as a mold.[21] Modern techniques generally involve placement of an expandable titanium cage from the posterolateral direction. The previously used Luque rectangles and sublaminar cables have been replaced by pedicle screws as the standard posterior fixation.

Lateral Extracavitary Approach

In the thoracic spine, lateral extracavitary approaches garnered greater interest prior to the era of transpedicular corpectomy.[14] For these approaches, the patient is positioned prone or three-quarters prone. The lesion is localized with preoperative fluoroscopy. "Hockey-stick" (midline "handle" with lateral "blade") or crescent-shaped incisions are surgical options. Skin and fascia are first opened at the midline. A lateral fascial incision at the injury level exposes the erector spinae, which are then elevated and retracted. The medial ribs, costotransverse joints, and costovertebral joints at the lesion level are dissected and cut/disarticulated. Removal of the rib requires careful dissection from the parietal pleura. Nerve roots are followed to the foramina. After removal of the ipsilateral pedicle, a vertebrectomy and diskectomy can be performed and the diseased level(s) addressed with the spinal cord under direct lateral visualization.[14] An expandable cage or other graft (including the harvested rib segment) can then be placed to reconstruct the anterior column. Finally, pedicle screws and rods can be placed from the same approach due to dorsal exposure and access. Unfortunately, the lateral extracavitary approach carries a high morbidity of up to 55% in the thoracic spine and might be best reserved for lesions inaccessible from other routes.

Transpedicular Corpectomy

For transpedicular corpectomies, pedicle screw insertion can be completed via an open, mini-open, or percutaneous technique.[22] In the open case, the fascia is fully opened, and paraspinal muscles fully dissected off the midline in the subperiosteal plane. They are retracted laterally to expose pedicle screw entry sites under direct visualization. For mini-open cases, skin is opened at the midline, but fascia is preserved. Pedicle screw placement then proceeds under either fluoroscopy or image-guidance with intraoperative O-arm CT scan.

For fluoroscopy-guided pedicle screw placement, Jamshidi needles are placed into the lateral margins of the pedicles under AP fluoroscopy guidance, using the same technique as for percutaneous screw placement. They are then advanced about 10 mm under AP guidance, taking care not to violate the pedicle medially or inferiorly. A lateral view is taken to ensure correct trajectory at this point. Again under AP guidance, the Jamshidi is advanced to 20 mm, and a lateral image then confirms whether the needle has passed through the posterior cortex of the vertebral body. Blunt-tip Kirschner wires (K-wires) are inserted into the Jamshidi needles and advanced to a depth of approximately 75% of the vertebral body. The Jamshidi is then removed and a cannulated pedicle screw is advanced over the K-wire. Extreme caution and frequent imaging should be used to avoid inadvertent ventral migration of the K-wire.

For image-guided pedicle screw placement, a single midline skin incision is made, again not opening the fascia. An intraoperative CT scan is performed with a reference marker on one of the caudal spinous processes. Then using intraoperative image navigation, a pilot hole is drilled with the navigated drill guide and drill. A navigated tap is used to prepare the entry site, and the appropriate screw size is measured. The pedicle screw is then advanced under navigation. Generally, three levels above and below the pathological vertebral body are instrumented, although two levels above and below can also be done in patients with excellent bone quality. It is critical to remember that rigid, durable fixation is essential for optimal pain relief and for preserving quality of life in patients with metastatic disease.

Although pedicle screws can be placed in a mini-open or percutaneous fashion, transpedicular corpectomy requires a midline fascial opening. Paraspinal muscles are dissected and retracted laterally to the rib. After laminectomy, the pedicle is removed with a rongeur or drill. Vertebrectomy is then performed using rongeurs and drills until reaching the anterior longitudinal ligament. A matchstick drill bit is recommended in order to minimize the risk to ventral tissues. Complete removal of the vertebra is not always necessary and depends on the surgical goals. Before completing the corpectomy, a temporary rod should be placed on the contralateral side. A Woodson or down-angle curette is used to dissect the posterior vertebral body off of the spinal cord or thecal sac and advance it ventrally.[21] The posterior vertebral body and posterior longitudinal ligament may contain tumor and should be removed. This is also necessary in order to achieve circumferential decompression.[21] The ipsilateral nerve root is ligated and transected preganglionically to create an entry path for the cage. The posterior longitudinal ligament is dissected free and opened, and the ventral and caudal disks are removed. Then a pathway along the rib head must be opened. The rib head can be removed or opened in a trapdoor fashion. The latter option avoids pleural dissection and the rib head can temporarily be swung open to allow placement of the cage.[23] A trial sizer should be placed to determine the largest possible safe cage placement. Finally, an expandable cage is passed into the corpectomy defect and expanded. The position is verified with an X-ray. Final rods and set screws are placed. In the open case, posterior arthrodesis is performed with auto- or allograft bone chips subjacent to the rod if life expectancy longer than 6 months is expected. An illustrative case is shown in **Figs. 6.1, 6.2, 6.3, 6.4, 6.5, 6.6**.

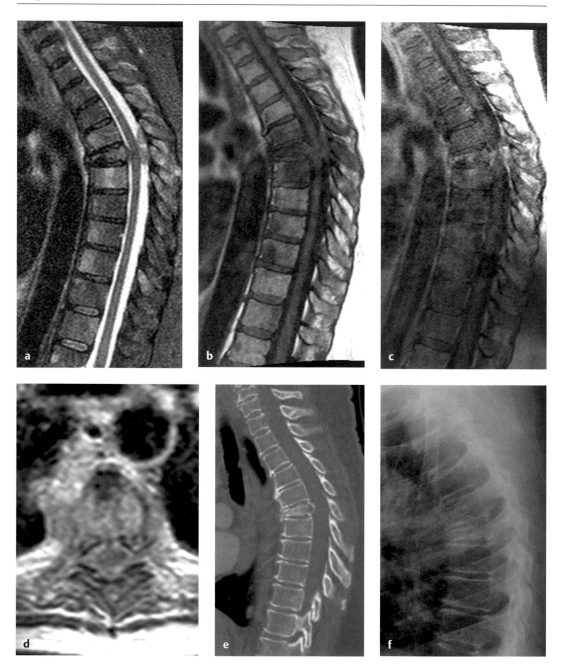

Fig. 6.1a–f Preoperative imaging in a 58-year-old woman with metastatic melanoma causing epidural spinal cord compression. The patient had an inability to ambulate and profound neurologic deficit. **(a)** Sagittal T2 magnetic resonance imaging (MRI) shows T6 pathological fracture with epidural spinal cord compression. **(b)** Sagittal T1 precontrast scan. **(c)** Postgadolinium T1 sagittal MRI scan shows enhancement in the T6 and T7 vertebral bodies as well as a posterior T6-7 enhancing mass lesion contributing to epidural spinal cord compression. **(d)** Axial T1 postgadolinium MRI scan at T6 shows circumferential epidural spinal cord compression. **(e)** Sagittal CT T-spine and **(f)** upright lateral chest X-ray scan better demonstrate the pathological collapse and kyphosis at T6.

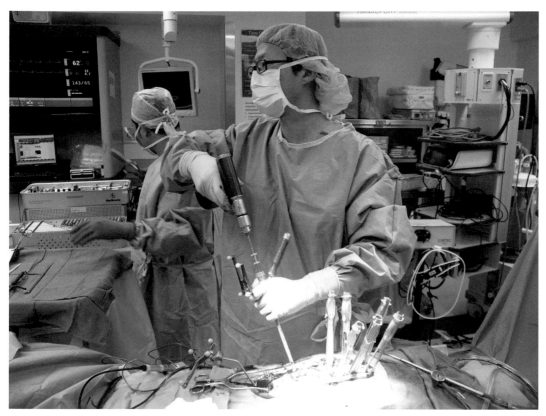

Fig. 6.2 Image-guided pedicle screw placement. The surgeon views the live monitor to verify correct trajectory while drilling a pilot hole. The drill guide is attached to infrared sensors (*four gray spheres on pink frame*) to determine its position in space. The fixed reference arc (*four gray spheres on blue frame*) is attached to a caudal spinous process prior to obtaining the intraoperative computed tomography (CT) scan.

In a single-institution study of 80 patients with thoracolumbar spine surgery, there was no difference in estimated blood loss (EBL), operative time, and complication rates when comparing single-level transpedicular with anterior-only corpectomies.[20] However, combined anterior-posterior corpectomies, had a higher complication rate, higher EBL, and increased operative time compared with the single-staged transpedicular corpectomy approach.

Lateral Approaches

True lateral approaches for vertebrectomy and reconstruction are particularly well suited to the midlumbar spine (L2-L4), where rib dissection is unnecessary and the iliac crest does not obstruct the surgical trajectory. Anterior reconstruction can be done from a lateral minimally invasive approach, and this is discussed in greater detail in Chapter 7.

Combined Approaches

Biomechanics

Combined anterior and posterior fixation may increase stiffness by approximately 50% compared with anterior cage placement and posterior fixation alone.[17] For anteriorly placed grafts or cages, posterior supplementation should almost always be considered when tumor invades the posterior elements, to provide necessary biomechanical instability, and to avoid late

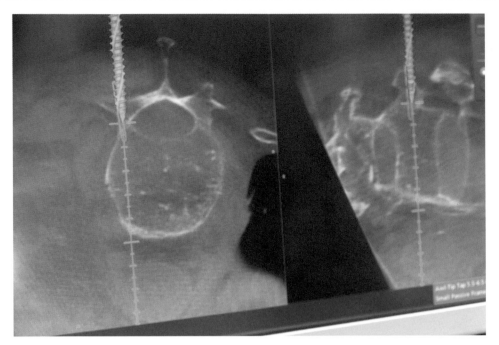

Fig. 6.3 Mini-open image-guided pedicle screw placement. After drilling a pilot hole, the pedicle and vertebral body are tapped under image navigation. Axial view is shown on the *left screen*. The *right screen* shows parasagittal view. The traversing pedicle tap (*violet*) and the current trajectory (*green hatched line*) are shown.

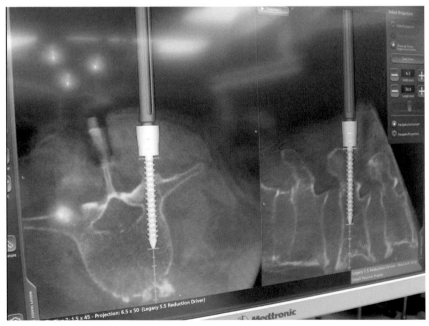

Fig. 6.4 Mini-open image-guided pedicle screw placement. After tapping the hole, the pedicle screw is advanced under image navigation. Axial view is shown on the *left screen*. The *right screen* shows parasagittal view. The traversing pedicle screw (*pink*), the screwdriver (*blue*), and the current trajectory (*green hatched line*) are shown.

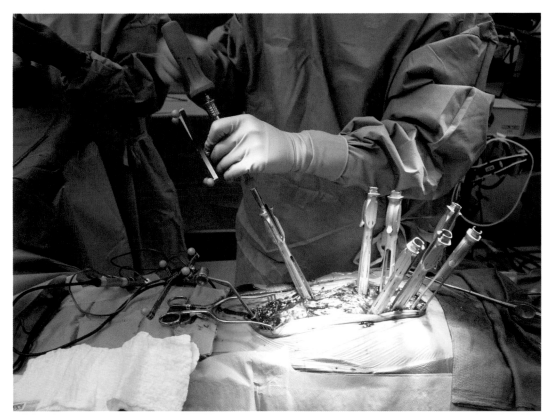

Fig. 6.5 Image-guided pedicle screw placement. The surgeon views the live monitor to determine the correct trajectory while advancing the pedicle screw. The screwdriver is attached to infrared sensors (*four gray spheres on dark gray frame*) to determine its position in space. The fixed reference arc (*four gray spheres on blue frame*) is attached to a caudal spinous process (*bottom left*).

construct failures. In cases of pathological kyphosis, junctional levels, or multiple adjacent vertebrectomies, posterior supplementation is essential.[5]

Posterior supplementation is more biomechanically stable than the native healthy motion segment or anterior fixation alone.[17,24] There is no biomechanical difference between static and expandable cages when combined with anterolateral vertebral body plating alone.[24] When combined with posterior supplementation, some studies found that expandable cages are more biomechanically stable for axial rotation, extension, and lateral bending than static mesh cages,[24] whereas others found no biomechanical difference.[17] Additionally, design variations in expandable cages do not appear to offer structural differences.[17]

Single-Stage Combined Approach

When tumor invades both anterior and posterior columns, combined approaches are often advantageous.[16,25] Lateral positioning is one option for such combined approaches to lesions at T5-L4 and offers the benefit of reduced intraabdominal pressure relative to prone positioning and simultaneous exposure for separate surgical teams working ventrally and dorsally.[25] Separate thoracotomy and midline thoracolumbar incisions are opened. If tumor extends to the ribs, these are transected laterally.[16] Laminectomies expose any epidural tumor, which is then dissected off of the dura or nerve roots. Segmental vessels are ligated to reduce vascular supply to the tumor, but not bilaterally in order to preserve spinal cord perfusion. Special

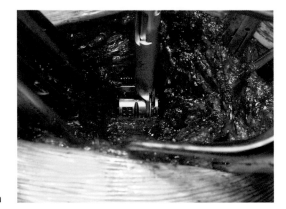

a

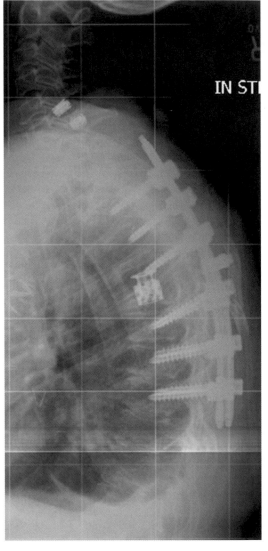

IN ST

Fig. 6.6a,b Postoperative imaging. Anteroposterior **(a)** and lateral **(b)** standing X-rays demonstrate good hardware placement. The expandable titanium cage is seen at the center of the construct. Pedicle screws were placed three levels above and below the level of the transpedicular corpectomy.

b

care must be taken near the artery of Adam-kiewicz. Ventral tissues and blood vessels are shifted away from the tumor. The spine must be stabilized posteriorly prior to performing the spondylectomy. Posterior instrumentation can be placed with the patient in the lateral position or the patient can be rotated prone if positioned on a mobile table with appropriate padding.[25] Removal of the pathological verte-bral body and surrounding tumor then pro-ceeds from posterior to anterior diagonally, near the pedicle, using a high-speed drill and ultra-sonic aspirator as needed.[4] The spinal cord or

thecal sac is decompressed circumferentially. In a retrospective study by Fourney et al, the anterior column was reconstructed with meth-ylmethacrylate using the chest tube technique, followed by placement of an anterior locking plate and screws.[16] Patients with metastatic spinal tumors survived a mean 22.5 months after surgery.[16] The presence of extraspinal me-tastasis was a predictor of a shorter survival (a mean of 17 months vs 47 months for no extraspinal metastasis); 62% of patients with preoperative neurologic deficit showed post-operative improvement, and 96% of patients had significant improvement in pain at 1 month follow-up, with the median visual analogue scale (VAS) pain score decreasing to zero at 1 year follow-up.[16]

■ Chapter Summary

For patients with spinal metastatic tumors, spine reconstruction and fixation/fusion can be performed from an anterior, posterior, lateral, or combined approach. For carefully selected patients with neurologic deficits related to tumor invasion, instability, and life expectancy of approximately three months, tumor resection combined with spine reconstruction affords improvements in neurologic function, pain, quality of life, and possibly longevity.[5] Anterior options include anterior cervical corpectomy, transthoracic corpectomy, and abdominal retroperitoneal lumbar corpectomy. Anterior reconstruction and plating are satisfactory in single-level, nonjunctional, and minimal deformity cases. Combined anterior and posterior fixation provides for the greatest biomechanical stiffness and stability.[17] Posterior options include extracavitary or transpedicular (posterolateral) corpectomy with expandable cage placement. The latter provides access for anterior column reconstruction and posterior instrumentation from a single approach. Tumors with both anterior and posterior involvement can be approached from a single posterolateral approach or single lateral position using a simultaneous combined approach.

Pearls

- Seventy percent of cases involve the thoracic spine, 20% the lumbar spine, and 10% the cervical spine, with most metastases going to the vertebral bodies rather than to the posterior elements.[8] The anatomic differences of each region necessitate different surgical approaches for surgical reconstruction and fusion (see Chapter 5 for further details).

- Circumferential surgical decompression with adjuvant radiotherapy is indicated for patients with metastatic epidural spinal cord compression, neurologic deficit (including pain), and expected survival of at least 3 months.[5] The minimum expected survival time needed to undergo surgery may shorten as minimally invasive techniques evolve.
- Hypervascular tumors should be assessed for preoperative embolization.
- Patients with metastatic spinal tumors may often have poor bone quality related to the primary cancer, poor nutritional status, and adjuvant chemotherapy and radiation.[9] It is thus imperative to reconstruct the spine with constructs of adequate biomechanical strength.
- In patients who undergo a destabilizing spondylectomy, options for vertebral body reconstruction include auto- or allograft bone, polymethylmethacrylate, static mesh cages, and expandable titanium cages.
- For anterior approaches to vertebral body reconstruction, posterior supplementation is advised for kyphotic lesions, junctional lesions, multilevel vertebrectomies, and in patients with extended life expectancy.
- For patients with metastatic spinal tumors, the goal of surgical reconstruction is generally palliative. Surgery should be planned to preserve neurologic function, alleviate pain, and correct instability.[16]

Pitfalls

- Patient's with poor overall functional state and significant comorbidities must not be operated on without careful preoperative evaluation. Patients who are poor candidates for spinal reconstruction with fixation and fusion may still qualify for percutaneous cement augmentation (see Chapter 8) or radiation therapy.
- Radiosensitive tumors such as lymphoma and myeloma may be best treated with radiation first,[6] if stability is not an issue.
- Anterior reconstruction without posterior supplementation is likely inadequate in cases of multilevel vertebrectomy, involvement of the cervicothoracic or thoracolumbar junction, significant kyphotic deformity, or tumor involvement of the posterior elements.
- Transpedicular corpectomy is highly destabilizing. At least two levels above and below the corpectomy should be instrumented, and a cross linker should be placed. In cases of poor bone quality, such as osteoporosis, three levels above and below are recommended.

References
Five Must-Read References

1. Bilsky MH, Lis E, Raizer J, Lee H, Boland P. The diagnosis and treatment of metastatic spinal tumor. Oncologist 1999;4:459–469
2. Young RF, Post EM, King GA. Treatment of spinal epidural metastases. Randomized prospective comparison of laminectomy and radiotherapy. J Neurosurg 1980;53:741–748
3. Black P. Spinal metastasis: current status and recommended guidelines for management. Neurosurgery 1979;5:726–746
4. Cybulski GR. Methods of surgical stabilization for metastatic disease of the spine. Neurosurgery 1989; 25:240–252
5. Patchell RA, Tibbs PA, Regine WF, et al. Direct decompressive surgical resection in the treatment of spinal cord compression caused by metastatic cancer: a randomised trial. Lancet 2005;366:643–648
6. Witham TF, Khavkin YA, Gallia GL, Wolinsky JP, Gokaslan ZL. Surgery insight: current management of epidural spinal cord compression from metastatic spine disease. Nat Clin Pract Neurol 2006;2:87–94, quiz 116
7. Bilsky MH, Boland P, Lis E, Raizer JJ, Healey JH. Single-stage posterolateral transpedicle approach for spondylectomy, epidural decompression, and circumferential fusion of spinal metastases. Spine 2000; 25:2240–2249, discussion 250
8. Gokaslan ZL, York JE, Walsh GL, et al. Transthoracic vertebrectomy for metastatic spinal tumors. J Neurosurg 1998;89:599–609
9. Viswanathan A, Abd-El-Barr MM, Doppenberg E, et al. Initial experience with the use of an expandable titanium cage as a vertebral body replacement in patients with tumors of the spinal column: a report of 95 patients. Eur Spine J 2012;21:84–92
10. De Giacomo T, Francioni F, Diso D, et al. Anterior approach to the thoracic spine. Interact Cardiovasc Thorac Surg 2011;12:692–695
11. Shufflebarger HL, Grimm JO, Bui V, Thomson JD. Anterior and posterior spinal fusion. Staged versus same-day surgery. Spine 1991;16:930–933
12. Passias PG, Ma Y, Chiu YL, Mazumdar M, Girardi FP, Memtsoudis SG. Comparative safety of simultaneous and staged anterior and posterior spinal surgery. Spine 2012;37:247–255
13. Wright N. Single-surgeon simultaneous versus staged anterior and posterior spinal reconstruction: a comparative study. J Spinal Disord Tech 2005;18(Suppl): S48–S57
14. Resnick DK, Benzel EC. Lateral extracavitary approach for thoracic and thoracolumbar spine trauma:

operative complications. Neurosurgery 1998;43:796–802, discussion 802–803
15. Charles YP, Barbe B, Beaujeux R, Boujan F, Steib JP. Relevance of the anatomical location of the Adamkiewicz artery in spine surgery. Surg Radiol Anat 2011;33:3–9
16. Fourney DR, Abi-Said D, Rhines LD, et al. Simultaneous anterior-posterior approach to the thoracic and lumbar spine for the radical resection of tumors followed by reconstruction and stabilization. J Neurosurg 2001;94(2, Suppl):232–244
17. Pflugmacher R, Schleicher P, Schaefer J, et al. Biomechanical comparison of expandable cages for vertebral body replacement in the thoracolumbar spine. Spine 2004;29:1413–1419
18. Lubelski D, Abdullah KG, Steinmetz MP, et al. Lateral extracavitary, costotransversectomy, and transthoracic thoracotomy approaches to the thoracic spine: review of techniques and complications. J Spinal Disord Tech 2013;26:222–232
19. Jandial R, Kelly B, Chen MY. Posterior-only approach for lumbar vertebral column resection and expandable cage reconstruction for spinal metastases. J Neurosurg Spine 2013;19:27–33
20. Lu DC, Lau D, Lee JG, Chou D. The transpedicular approach compared with the anterior approach: an analysis of 80 thoracolumbar corpectomies. J Neurosurg Spine 2010;12:583–591
21. Akeyson EW, McCutcheon IE. Single-stage posterior vertebrectomy and replacement combined with posterior instrumentation for spinal metastasis. J Neurosurg 1996;85:211–220
22. Lu DC, Chou D, Mummaneni PV. A comparison of mini-open and open approaches for resection of thoracolumbar intradural spinal tumors. J Neurosurg Spine 2011;14:758–764
23. Chou D, Wang VY. Trap-door rib-head osteotomies for posterior placement of expandable cages after transpedicular corpectomy: an alternative to lateral extracavitary and costotransversectomy approaches. J Neurosurg Spine 2009;10:40–45
24. Knop C, Lange U, Bastian L, Blauth M. Three-dimensional motion analysis with Synex. Comparative biomechanical test series with a new vertebral body replacement for the thoracolumbar spine. Eur Spine J 2000;9:472–485
25. Peeling L, Frangou E, Hentschel S, Gokaslan ZL, Fourney DR. Refinements to the simultaneous anterior-posterior approach to the thoracolumbar spine. J Neurosurg Spine 2010;12:456–461

7

Minimally Invasive Surgery for Metastatic Spine Disease

Meic H. Schmidt

■ Introduction

Minimally invasive treatment (MIT) of spinal tumors is becoming increasingly complex, and multiple specialties are contributing to bring their techniques to the fore.[1] These modalities include percutaneous techniques (e.g., image-guided biopsy, embolization, cement augmentation, radiofrequency ablation) and minimally invasive surgery (MIS) techniques. Current MIS techniques are key components of MIT for the treatment of metastatic spine disease.

This chapter defines MIS, discusses the MIS techniques that can be used in addition to traditional open techniques, examines potential criteria for the use and evaluation of MIS techniques, and provides an overview of posterior and anterior surgical MIS techniques, focusing on the thoracoscopic approach for tumor resection via corpectomy, followed by reconstruction and stabilization.

■ What Is Minimally Invasive?

Although a precise definition of the term *minimally invasive* is elusive, most authors agree that MIS involves surgical techniques that reduce collateral tissue damage most commonly associated with surgical access (approach).[2] MIS can potentially decrease access-associated mor-bidity such as postoperative wound infection, reduce the need for blood transfusion, and enable faster recovery by allowing for earlier postoperative adjuvant treatment (e.g., radiation, chemotherapy).

Minimally invasive surgery can also entail doing less surgery at the target site under the principle that "less is more." If a better outcome would be expected from adjuvant treatment after an initial surgery, that option should be considered. For example, decompressing the spinal cord without removing all the tumor tissue might be sufficient if the patient is a suitable candidate for radiation after surgery.[3] In that sense, MIS can entail doing less surgery to achieve the equivalent or better outcome compared with more extensive surgical resection. For example, Laufer et al[3] recently published a series of 186 patients treated with "separation surgery" followed by adjuvant hypofractionated or high-dose single-fraction radiosurgery. Although minimal access techniques were not used in this series, "separation surgery" conceptually shows that less surgery can achieve equal or better results for palliative care of metastatic spine disease. It involves decompression of the thecal sac by a limited posterior lateral tumor resection and posterior segmental instrumentation, followed by postoperative cytotoxic radiosurgery doses that spare the spinal cord. The results show that local tumor control was achieved in the majority of patients, with a cumulative incidence of local progression 1 year after radiosurgery of 16.4%. Only four patients required reoperation.

Thus, it is difficult to reach a consensus on a definition of MIS, which can have different meanings for different authors. It is similarly difficult to define the added value of MIS based on quality and cost measures. The Text Box lists some of the criteria I use to evaluate and justify MIS procedures including those undertaken for metastatic spine disease. Although by no means a complete list, these criteria can be used to analyze and compare various surgical approaches including open, mini-open, endoscopic, and percutaneous techniques.

Criteria for minimally invasive spine surgery to be meaningful and valuable

1. Minimizing surgically induced tissue damage
   a. Smaller, cosmetically appealing skin incision
   b. Minimal muscle dissection
   c. Less bone removal
2. Measurable clinical benefit
   a. Decrease in surgical morbidity and mortality
      i. Cerebrospinal fluid leak, neurologic worsening, less instability
   b. Lower intraoperative blood loss
      i. Less need for blood transfusion
      ii. Less need for cell saver
   c. Shorter stay in the hospital
      i. Fewer days in intensive care unit
      ii. Shorter overall stay
      iii. Lower readmission rate
   d. Resumption of activities
      i. Less need for rehabilitation
      ii. Less need for physical therapy
      iii. Faster return to work
   e. Lower infection rates
   f. Lower reoperation rates
   g. Earlier initiation of postoperative therapies
      i. Physical therapy, radiation, chemotherapy
3. Clinical effectiveness
   a. MIS must achieve the intended surgical goal
      i. Decompression, reconstruction
   b. MIS must have equivalent or better clinical outcomes
      i. Neurologic improvement and pain outcome
   c. MIS must have equivalent or better imaging outcomes
      i. Fusion rate
      ii. Spinal canal decompression

4. Favorable socioeconomic effect
   a. MIS must improve quality
      i. Increase in quality measures listed above (criteria 1–3)
   b. MIS must be cost effective
      i. Upfront cost must be balanced with downstream cost savings
      ii. Imaging cost associated with MIS
   c. MIS must be valuable
      i. Value = quality/cost

■ Posterior and Posterolateral Approaches

Posterior surgical approaches are used for laminectomies and transpedicular decompression. More extensive posterolateral approaches like the lateral extracavitary approach allow for extensive posterior and anterior decompression including more complete corpectomy and en bloc resection.[4] Because of the extensive soft tissue trauma associated with these traditional approaches, MIS techniques were developed to take advantage of the access trajectory of the approaches by minimizing the incision.[5–7]

Deutsch et al[6] applied the MIS technique using a tubular retractor to access spinal metastasis to the thoracic spine in eight patients (**Fig. 7.1**). Through unilateral or bilateral 3-cm incisions they performed intralesional, transpedicular vertebrectomies for spinal cord decompression with limited reconstruction using methylmethacrylate. None of the patients underwent spinal stabilization using instrumentation. The mean operative time and mean blood loss were 2.2 hours and 270 mL, respectively. The mean length of stay was 4 days. Postoperatively, 62.5% of patients had improved neurologic function and pain control. All patients underwent postoperative radiation therapy. No complications related to surgery were noted.

Zairi et al[7] described 10 patients with metastasis to the thoracic spine who were treated with decompressive corpectomy using a tubular retractor. No anterior column reconstruction was performed after transpedicular corpectomy;

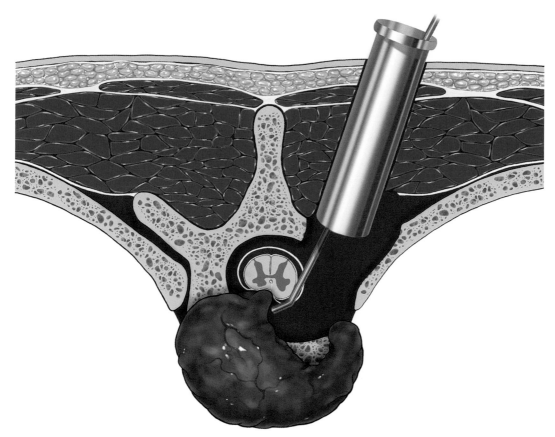

Fig. 7.1 Illustration of exposure for minimally invasive transpedicular vertebrectomy. The tubular retractor facilitates the lateral exposure so that the anterior portion of the spine can be visualized. (Courtesy of the Department of Neurosurgery, University of Utah.)

however, the authors used percutaneous pedicle screw fixation to stabilize the spine (**Fig. 7.2**). They reported a mean operative time of 170 minutes and mean estimated blood loss of 400 mL. No patient required a blood transfusion. The mean length of stay was 6 days. The only complication reported was a postoperative urinary tract infection. Eighty percent of patients improved by at least one Frankel grade.

Both series demonstrated excellent radiographic and clinical results but involved only a small number of patients. It is important to note that in both series patients with overt neoplastic spinal instability (i.e., kyphosis) were excluded. A major disadvantage of any approach with a posterior incision is the risk of infection, which is particularly high in cancer patients, who are frequently immunocompromised and have often had prior radiation therapy. Infection can be a life-threatening event in oncology because of the limited capacity of patients to fight it despite antibiotic therapy. In addition, infections frequently disqualify patients from adjuvant radiation, chemotherapy, and experimental protocols. Prior studies indicate that the risk of a posterior wound infection in a cancer patient is approximately 12 to 32%, depending on the timing of radiation.[8] These initial studies on posterior MIS techniques in cancer patients have not yet clearly demonstrated a lower infection risk compared with standard open posterior and anterior approaches.

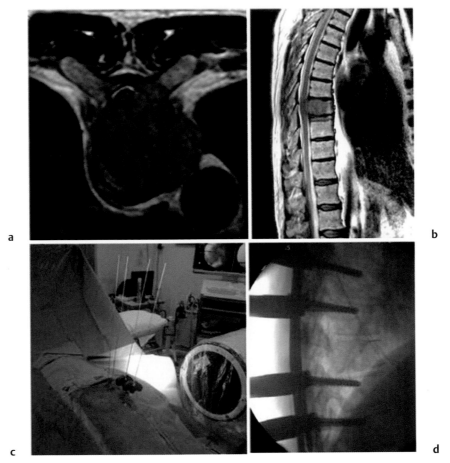

Fig. 7.2a–d Axial **(a)** and sagittal **(b)** T2-weighted magnetic resonance imaging (MRI) depicting spinal cord compression due to a metastasis at T7. **(c)** The operative photograph shows insertion of the wires on the right side. **(d)** Lateral fluoroscopy shows the spine after bilateral pedicle screw insertion and the introduction of the rods. (From Zairi F, Arikat A, Allaoui M, Marinho P, Assaker R. Minimally invasive decompression and stabilization for the management of thoracolumbar spine metastasis. J Neurosurg Spine 2012;17(1):21. Reproduced with permission.)

■ Anterior and Anterolateral Approaches

Traditional Thoracotomy

Although resection of metastatic spine tumors was historically performed via a posterior laminectomy approach, it frequently resulted in unsatisfactory outcome and neurologic worsening. The most common reason for therapeutic failure is related to the fact that most metastases originate in the vertebral body and are associated with a degree of spinal instability that can be worsened by an indirect decompression with a simple laminectomy. At the same time, anterior open thoracotomy and thoracoabdominal approaches were demonstrating improved outcomes by more effectively addressing the goals of tumor resection, neural decompression, and anterior reconstruction. Transpleural thoracotomy allows for direct access to the spinal canal for decompression, anterior column reconstruction, and stabilization. Thoracotomy can be extended to include the upper lumbar spine by incising the diaphragm (thoracolumbar approach).

Several published case series document the excellent outcomes of thoracotomy for pain control, neurologic improvement, and spinal stability for metastatic disease. Gokaslan et al[9] reported one of the largest series of patients who underwent traditional thoracotomy for metastatic disease at M.D. Anderson. Seventy-two patients with metastatic spine tumors underwent thoracotomy for transthoracic vertebrectomy, decompression, reconstruction with polymethyl methacrylate, and anterior plate fixation; supplemental posterior fixation was used in seven patients. The study found that 76% of patients had improved neurologic function and 77% of nonambulatory patients regained the ability to walk. Spinal pain decreased in 92.3% (60/65) of patients who initially presented with pain. It is important to note that pain was assessed at 1-month follow-up to allow incisional pain to resolve. Although the risk of wound infection in this series was < 1% (a fraction of the infection risk compared with any posterior incision surgery), the morbidity related to thoracotomy access, including postthoracotomy pain, was approximately 17%. In many patients, the postthoracotomy pain was severe enough to require narcotics for pain control.

Because these thoracotomy techniques still involved access morbidity, several MIS techniques for anterior access have been developed for spine surgery (**see Text Box**).

Minimally Invasive Surgery Approaches and Techniques for Metastatic Spine Disease

◆ Posterior/posterolateral
  ○ Percutaneous/mini-open pedicle screw fixation
  ○ Tubular access for decompression
◆ Anterior/anterolateral
  ○ Mini-open thoracotomy (transpleural, retropleural)
  ○ Video-assisted thoracoscopic surgery

Mini-thoracotomy and thoracoscopic approaches have been used in cardiothoracic surgery to minimize the access morbidity, and over the years both techniques have been ad-opted for spine pathologies such as thoracic disk herniation, spine fracture, and tumors. The goal of both anterior MIS techniques is to decrease the access morbidity without compromising the safety and efficacy of the spinal procedure to be performed. At the target disease site, the MIS technique needs to enable a corpectomy to decompress the spinal canal, followed by interbody reconstruction and stabilization.

Mini-Open Thoracotomy

Current anterior mini-open MIS approaches use either a retropleural or transpleural approach. Most patient series are small and retrospective evaluations, but they demonstrate the feasibility of the mini-open approach. Huang et al[10] reported a retrospective series of 46 patients with spine metastases: 29 underwent mini-thoracotomy and 17 underwent standard thoracotomy for anterior corpectomy and reconstruction. Clinical and surgical outcomes were similar with the two techniques; however, only 6.9% of mini-thoracotomy patients required a stay as long as 2 days in the intensive care unit compared with 88% of the standard thoracotomy group. Uribe et al[11] reported their experience of a mini-open retropleural approach for thoracic tumor removal in 21 patients, although the majority of tumors were not metastatic but rather other primary intra- and extradural lesions. Operating time, estimated blood loss, and length of stay were 117 minutes, 291 mL, and 2.9 days, respectively.

I prefer to use a table-mounted retractor system for mini-open thoracotomy (SynFrame, DePuy Synthes, West Chester, PA). Payer and Sottas[12] reported a case series of 37 patients in whom the SynFrame was used. Eleven patients had metastatic spine lesions. The mean operating time and mean blood loss were 188 minutes and 711 mL, respectively. Two patients had complications. Neurologic and pain improvement were excellent.

The major advantage of the mini-open thoracotomy is that it enables the surgeon to use the microscope or loupes for a three-dimensional view of the spine. In addition, the lung does not need to be deflated or at least can be partially ventilated during surgery. Disadvantages of the

Table 7.1 Thoracoscopic Vertebrectomy

Study	Total Number of Procedures/ Number of Procedures for Tumor	Types of Fixation Used	Mean Operating Room Time	Mean Estimated Blood Loss (mL)	Mean Duration of Chest Tube Use (Days)	Mean Length of Hospital Stay (Days)
McAfee et al (1995)[13]	15 VBR, 8 tumors	NA	211 min	890 (150–2,800)	1.22 (1–3)	6.5 (2–12)
Rosenthal et al (1996)[15]	28 VBR, 4 tumors	PMMA, Z plate	6.8 h	1,450	NA	NA
Dickman et al (1996)[14]	17 VBR, 7 tumors	PMMA, Z plate	347 min	1,117	2.8	8.7

Abbreviations: VBR, thoracoscopic vertebrectomy; NA, not available; PMMA, polymethylmethacrylate.

mini-open approach are the relatively longer incision and the partial removal of the rib that is necessary. This rib resection can cause pain in the postoperative period and can affect the patient's ability to breathe. Another disadvantage of the mini-open technique is the difficulty with using appropriate surgical tools. Because of the long working distance from the chest wall to the spine, many traditional micro-tools are too short. In addition, many tools used for thoracoscopic surgery are too long to fit under the microscope easily and they interfere with direct visualization of the target site. This problem can be circumvented by either using surgical loupes or a microscope with long focal length. Alternatively, a hybrid technique using both loupes and the endoscope, which gives more room to use longer tools, can be employed.

Thoracoscopic techniques have been used by thoracic surgeons for many years to avoid thoracotomy-related access morbidity of traditional open and mini-open thoracotomy. Thoracoscopy has been adapted for use in spinal surgery for the treatment of thoracic disk herniations and traumatic fractures. Three series illustrated that thoracoscopy can be applied to spine surgery including corpectomy (**Table 7.1**).[13–15] The major shortcoming described by all of the authors was the limited ability to perform without difficulty an instrumented stabilization after thoracoscopic corpectomy and an interbody reconstruction. To address this difficulty, Beisse[16] pioneered an endoscopic anterolateral plating system that could be placed via small thoracoscopic port incisions. My group

at the Huntsman Cancer Institute and the University of Utah (Salt Lake City, Utah) has slightly modified the MIS thoracoscopic technique for metastatic spine tumors.[17–23]

■ Minimally Invasive Surgery Using the Thoracoscopic Approach

As with other endoscopic procedures, access to the thoracic cavity is achieved using small chest incisions for access portals, and the surgery is performed with specially designed instruments. By using small thoracoscopic incisions, which minimize chest wall dissection and retraction, postoperative morbidity has been significantly reduced by decreasing blood loss, postoperative pain, pulmonary and shoulder dysfunction, days in the intensive care unit, and overall hospital stay. Since its inception, minimally invasive thoracoscopic surgery has improved significantly with the advancement of endoscopic video technology and the development of surgical tools and anterior plating systems. Many procedures that had previously been performed via open thoracotomy can now be performed safely and effectively with the minimally invasive thoracoscopic approach.

Thoracoscopic spinal surgery is an alternative MIS technique to traditional thoracotomy for tumor and vertebral body resection, thoracic corpectomy, anterior neural decompression, and anterolateral spinal reconstruction.

The goals of surgery are to resect tumor and diseased vertebral body, decompress the anterior spinal canal, and restore biomechanical stability with interbody reconstruction augmented with anterolateral plating.

Preoperative Planning

A good understanding of the general regional and individual patient anatomy of the thoracolumbar spine, spinal cord, chest wall and thorax, and mediastinal structures is important when planning for thoracoscopic surgery. The side of surgery is chosen based on the location and lateralization of disease in relation to the surrounding anatomy (e.g., the aorta). In general, a left-sided approach is used for the thoracolumbar junction (T11-L2) and for disease on the left side. A right-sided approach is preferred for the middle to upper thoracic spine (T3-10). Because of the potential vascular complication from thoracic anterior lateral instrumentation, my group chooses the side away from the aorta.

The bony anatomy is studied preoperatively to plan the reconstruction. The vertebral body widths are measured to determine the length of the posterolateral vertebral body screws. The extent of resection, or the distance between the inferior end plate of the cranial level and the superior end plate of the caudal level, is also measured to determine the size of the interbody implant. In addition, we note the potential bone quality, including factors such as osteoporosis and other metastatic lytic lesions in the adjacent vertebral bodies.

Technique

Thoracoscopic surgery requires a high-quality endoscopic camera, which is essential for optimal illumination and visualization. Endoscopic instruments are designed with nonreflective surfaces for decreased glare, are of adequate length for safe intrathoracic maneuvering, and have large handles for ease of use. Specialized instrumentation for thoracoscopic spinal reconstruction has also been developed. The MACS-TL (Modular Anterior Construct System for the Thoracic and Lumbar Spine) anterolateral spinal implant (Aesculap, Tuttlingen, Germany) is a rigid fixation plate specifically designed for endoscopic use, differing from most other thoracolumbar plating systems, which have been developed for open surgery.

Thoracoscopic spine surgery is performed with the patient under general anesthesia and single-lung ventilation, which provides maximum surgical exposure. Whereas mini-open MIS approaches can be performed without single lung ventilation, it is nearly impossible to do this with thoracoscopy.

The patient is placed in a lateral decubitus position with the spine parallel to a radiolucent operating table, with the side of surgery chosen preoperatively based on the patient's anatomy (**Fig. 7.3a,b**). After the patient is positioned optimally, a lateral spine view is obtained using the C-arm fluoroscope to determine the relation of the spine and access portals. The involved vertebral bodies, intervertebral disks, anterior and posterior spinal lines, and four portal access sites are then marked on the skin. Proper positioning of these portals enables the optimal use of the camera retractors and tools (**Fig. 7.3c**).

The entire area of the lateral chest wall is sterilized and draped to prepare for possible conversion to open thoracotomy. The portal located in the most cranial direction is opened first to minimize the risk of injury to the diaphragm and underlying organs. After the skin incision is made, the opening is carried down to the rib using a mini-thoracotomy technique. The subcutaneous tissues and intercostal muscle layers are freed from the rib using a blunt dissection technique without removing any rib to minimize injury to the underlying lung. In comparison to traditional and most mini-open approaches, the removal of the rib is not necessary, which eliminates a source of postoperative pain. The first trocar is then inserted, and the 30-degree endoscope is used to inspect the thoracic cavity. The remaining three ports are inserted directly under thoracoscopic vision.

When operating at or below the insertion, the diaphragm is incised to expose the spine. The prevertebral soft tissue dissection is performed next for exposure of the thoracic vertebral bodies and intervertebral disks. The correct

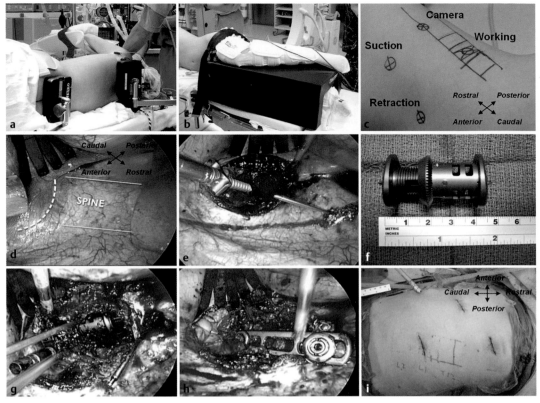

Fig. 7.3a–i **(a–c)** Intraoperative photographs depicting positioning. **(d,e,g,h)** Key endoscopic views. **(f)** Hardware. **(i)** Closure. **(a)** The patient is positioned on a radiolucent table in the right lateral decubitus position for a left-sided thoracoscopic approach to L1. The independent arm is in a Krause frame. Adjustable pads at the pubis, sternum, and lower and upper spine hold the patient in position. **(b)** The independent leg is slightly flexed at the hip to facilitate iliopsoas relaxation, making it easier to dissect this muscle off the lateral aspect of the vertebral bodies at the thoracolumbar junction. **(c)** The level of interest is marked, identifying the vertebral body above and below, and the four chest portals are planned. **(d)** Endoscopic view of the spine (*solid lines*). The diaphragm is swept inferiorly with a fan retractor and a diaphragmatic incision is planned (*dotted lines*). **(e)** A Kirschner wire is placed above the planned corpectomy and a polyaxial screw-clamp combination is placed below it. **(f)** Lateral view of a fully expanded gear-driven cage. **(g)** The cage is placed and expanded within the central corpectomy. **(h)** Final anterolateral plate construct. **(i)** Closure with chest tube exiting the retraction port. (From Ragel BT, Amini A, Schmidt MH. Thoracoscopic vertebral body replacement with an expandable cage after ventral spinal canal decompression. Neurosurgery 2007;61(5 Suppl 2):ONS319. Reproduced with permission.)

level is identified visually. After completion of the exposure, the surgeon proceeds with placement of the vertebral body screws, which is followed by tumor resection, decompression, and reconstruction (**Fig. 7.3d,e**).

In the thoracoscopic approach, it is advantageous to place the vertebral body screws above and below the corpectomy prior to the resection. One of the disadvantages of thoracoscopy is the lack of three-dimensional vision, and the screws can be used to maintain proper orientation in a two-dimensional surgical field. The clamps of the screws are attached to the screw heads so that they are oriented parallel to the end plates with the holes for the stabilizing screws situated anteriorly. These screws define

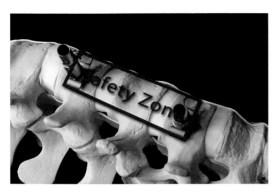

Fig. 7.4 The borders of the clamps define a safety zone and the extent of corpectomy. The resection is performed within these safe boundaries. (From Bishop FS, Schmidt MH. Thoracoscopic resection and reconstruction. In: Ames C, Boriani, Jandial R, eds. Spine and Spinal Cord Tumors: Advanced Management and Operative Techniques. St. Louis: Quality Medical Publishing, 2013. Reproduced with permission.)

the anteromedial and posterolateral borders of an area that includes both the extent of corpectomy and a safety zone that protects critical structures. The resection is performed by keeping instruments within these safe boundaries (**Fig. 7.4**).

The diskectomies are performed endoscopically at the disk spaces above and below the lesion, similarly to an open procedure. Decompression of the spinal canal is necessary for tumors extending past the posterior vertebral body wall. Tumor and bone fragments in the epidural space are carefully brought into the corpectomy cavity and removed. The resection is complete when gross tumor is removed, the anterior spinal canal is decompressed, and the corpectomy adequately accommodates the interbody device.

After tumor resection, spinal cord decompression, and corpectomy, my group prefers to use an expandable titanium cage for an anterolateral vertebral body reconstruction (**Fig. 7.3f,g**). Once it has been inserted, the cage is expanded with endoscopic and fluoroscopic visualization, noting its position in the coronal and sagittal planes. Fitting and securing the anterolateral plate completes the reconstruction

(**Fig. 7.3h**). The final construct position is verified with anteroposterior and lateral fluoroscopic imaging.

Closure of the operative site begins with reapproximation of the diaphragm if it was opened. The thoracic cavity is inspected for hemostasis and irrigated, removing visible blood clots. A 24-French chest tube is inserted under endoscopic visualization through the more ventrally located lung/diaphragm retractor portal or the suction/irrigation portal. The lung is reinflated and inspected with endoscopy to ensure that all lobes are properly inflated. The trocars are removed and the incisions are closed in multiple layers (**Fig. 7.3i**).

Postoperative computed tomography (CT) scans and plain radiographs centered on the construct are obtained, and patient mobilization and incentive spirometry training also begin on postoperative day 1. The chest tube is removed once the output decreases below 100 mL/day and the chest radiograph continues to demonstrate lung inflation without pneumothorax, typically on postoperative day 2. After removal of the chest tube, a final chest radiograph is used to verify stable lung inflation.

Results

Operative results for the minimally invasive thoracoscopic approach have demonstrated its efficacy and safety and are generally better than those associated with open surgery.[17,21–23] Operative times initially increase to an average of 6 hours or longer while the surgeon and operating room staff learn the new technique; however, the learning curve associated with thoracoscopic surgery can be overcome without additional morbidity to the patient.[23] The duration of surgery for tumor resection and reconstruction is decreased to 4 hours for the entire procedure after the technique has been mastered. The estimated blood loss has been reported to be 600 mL in thoracoscopic tumor cases, compared with 1 L during an open thoracotomy.[9,17,21] With care, intraoperative complications such as uncontrollable bleeding, cerebrospinal fluid or chyle leak, or injuries to the vessels or viscera can largely be avoided.

The rate of conversion to an open procedure, in skilled hands and with meticulous adherence to surgical technique, is ≤ 1%.[23]

The principal advantages of thoracoscopic surgery are the favorable clinical outcomes.[17,22] The overall morbidity is low, primarily because of the limited surgical exposure and approach. Although the morbidity rate for all open thoracotomy procedures is 14 to 29.5%, with tumor cases having a higher incidence than other open procedures, the complication rate of the thoracoscopic procedure is 0 to 5.4%. Reported complications include persistent pleural effusion, pneumonia, intercostal neuralgia, shoulder dysfunction, and transient L1 root deficit. Furthermore, open thoracotomy for tumor has a reported mortality of 8.2%, whereas no mortality has been reported for the thoracoscopic approach. Infection rates are low for both thoracotomy and thoracoscopic surgery, around 0.5%.

Patients experience a significant reduction in pain postoperatively with minimally invasive thoracoscopic surgery.[17] Duration and dosages of postoperative analgesic therapy have been reported to decrease by 31% and 42%, respectively.[16] Rates of chronic postoperative pain after thoracoscopic surgery are between 4% and 35%, which compares favorably with reported rates of 7 to 55% for open thoracotomy. The median length of stay in the hospital was 7 days (range, 4–10 days) in a series of patients who underwent thoracoscopic tumor surgery, compared with a median of 9 days (range, 4–57 days) for patients who underwent open thoracotomy for tumor resection.[9,17]

The learning curve for MIS procedures can be less difficult to overcome than is frequently reported.[23] Acquiring the techniques should be done progressively from open techniques to mini-open and closed techniques such as endoscopy and percutaneous procedures. In addition, the surgeon should not hesitate to convert to a mini-open or open procedure from a closed technique if the conditions warrant it. In my experience, it is much better to convert to a mini-open from a thoracoscopy approach than to spend hours to force a thoracoscopic procedure that is not going well. Unexpected findings and technical difficulties can be encountered that make an alternate approach better. In that sense, not every open conversion is a complication, but instead represents good judgment.

■ Chapter Summary

The role of MIS approaches for metastatic spine disease continues to evolve. The learning process for most MIS techniques can be mastered without exposing the patient to additional risk. Many MIS procedures are a smaller version of open techniques that a surgeon can incorporate with progressive experience. This is particularly true for posterior and posterolateral approaches. The use of endoscopy in MIS is somewhat more challenging because of the loss of three-dimensional vision. Clinical results for MIS in metastatic spine disease are comparable or better than traditional approaches. MIS approaches have become an important part in the management of metastatic spine disease, but their meaningful use and value have not been conclusively proven. Future studies will need to demonstrate in more detail the clinical and socioeconomic benefit.

Pearls

Minimally Invasive Surgery Thoracoscopic Technique
◆ If single-lung ventilation cannot be obtained, it is better to convert to a mini-open MIS approach.
◆ If a port is not in the optimal position, it is better to place a new port to optimize use of the camera and the endoscopic tools.
◆ Placement of the screws establishes visual reference points in a two-dimensional environment and helps to maintain orientation during thoracoscopic surgery.

Pitfall

Preoperative Planning of a Thoracoscopic Approach
◆ Operating on the side with the aorta overlying the spine is possible, but contact between the hardware and the large vessel can cause catastrophic injury in the long term and should be avoided.

Acknowledgments

The author thanks Kristin Kraus, MSc, for editorial assistance. The author is a consultant for Aesculap, Germany. Portions of this chapter were based on the chapter by Bishop and Schmidt.[18]

References

Five Must-Read References

1. Niazi TN, Sauri-Barraza JC, Schmidt MH. Minimally invasive treatment of spinal tumors. Semin Spine Surg 2011;23:51–59
2. McAfee PC, Phillips FM, Andersson G, et al. Minimally invasive spine surgery. Spine 2010;35(26, Suppl): S271–S273
3. Laufer I, Iorgulescu JB, Chapman T, et al. Local disease control for spinal metastases following "separation surgery" and adjuvant hypofractionated or high-dose single-fraction stereotactic radiosurgery: outcome analysis in 186 patients. J Neurosurg Spine 2013; 18:207–214
4. Schmidt MH, Larson SJ, Maiman DJ. The lateral extracavitary approach to the thoracic and lumbar spine. Neurosurg Clin N Am 2004;15:437–441
5. Lidar Z, Lifshutz J, Bhattacharjee S, Kurpad SN, Maiman DJ. Minimally invasive, extracavitary approach for thoracic disc herniation: technical report and preliminary results. Spine J 2006;6:157–163
6. Deutsch H, Boco T, Lobel J. Minimally invasive transpedicular vertebrectomy for metastatic disease to the thoracic spine. J Spinal Disord Tech 2008;21: 101–105
7. Zairi F, Arikat A, Allaoui M, Marinho P, Assaker R. Minimally invasive decompression and stabilization for the management of thoracolumbar spine metastasis. J Neurosurg Spine 2012;17:19–23
8. Ghogawala Z, Mansfield FL, Borges LF. Spinal radiation before surgical decompression adversely affects outcomes of surgery for symptomatic metastatic spinal cord compression. Spine 2001;26:818–824
9. Gokaslan ZL, York JE, Walsh GL, et al. Transthoracic vertebrectomy for metastatic spinal tumors. J Neurosurg 1998;89:599–609
10. Huang TJ, Hsu RW, Li YY, Cheng CC. Minimal access spinal surgery (MASS) in treating thoracic spine metastasis. Spine 2006;31:1860–1863
11. Uribe JS, Dakwar E, Le TV, Christian G, Serrano S, Smith WD. Minimally invasive surgery treatment for thoracic spine tumor removal: a mini-open, lateral approach. Spine 2010;35(26, Suppl):S347–S354
12. Payer M, Sottas C. Mini-open anterior approach for corpectomy in the thoracolumbar spine. Surg Neurol 2008;69:25–31, discussion 31–32
13. McAfee PC, Regan JR, Fedder IL, Mack MJ, Geis WP. Anterior thoracic corpectomy for spinal cord decompression performed endoscopically. Surg Laparosc Endosc 1995;5:339–348
14. Dickman CA, Rosenthal D, Karahalios DG, et al. Thoracic vertebrectomy and reconstruction using a microsurgical thoracoscopic approach. Neurosurgery 1996;38:279–293
15. Rosenthal D, Marquardt G, Lorenz R, Nichtweiss M. Anterior decompression and stabilization using a microsurgical endoscopic technique for metastatic tumors of the thoracic spine. J Neurosurg 1996;84: 565–572
16. Beisse R. Endoscopic surgery on the thoracolumbar junction of the spine. Eur Spine J 2010;19(Suppl 1): S52–S65
17. Kan P, Schmidt MH. Minimally invasive thoracoscopic approach for anterior decompression and stabilization of metastatic spine disease. Neurosurg Focus 2008;25:E8
18. Bishop FS, Schmidt MH. Thoracoscopic resection and reconstruction. In: Ames C, Boriani, Jandial R, eds. Spine and Spinal Cord Tumors: Advanced Management and Operative Techniques. St. Louis: Quality Medical Publishing, 2013:607–628
19. Bishop FS, Schmidt MH. Thoracoscopic corpectomy, interbody reconstruction and stabilization. In: Benzel E, ed. Spine Surgery: Techniques, Complication Avoidance, 3rd ed. Philadelphia: Elsevier Churchill Livingstone, 2012:583–592
20. Ragel BT, Amini A, Schmidt MH. Thoracoscopic vertebral body replacement with an expandable cage after ventral spinal canal decompression. Neurosurgery 2007;61(5, Suppl 2):317–322, discussion 322–323
21. Ragel BT, Kan P, Schmidt MH. Blood transfusions after thoracoscopic anterior thoracolumbar vertebrectomy. Acta Neurochir (Wien) 2010;152:597–603
22. Ray WZ, Krisht KM, Dailey AT, Schmidt MH. Clinical outcomes of unstable thoracolumbar junction burst fractures: combined posterior short-segment correction followed by thoracoscopic corpectomy and fusion. Acta Neurochir (Wien) 2013;155:1179–1186
23. Ray WZ, Schmidt MH. Thoracoscopic vertebrectomy for thoracolumbar junction fractures and tumors: Surgical technique and evaluation of the learning curve. J Spinal Disord Tech 2013; in press

8

Vertebral Augmentation for Metastatic Disease

Ehud Mendel, Eric C. Bourekas, and Paul Porensky

▪ Introduction

Percutaneous vertebroplasty (PVP) is an effective and relatively facile intervention that can achieve both vertebral stabilization and augmentation. This technique, first described for the treatment of painful hemangiomas, has expanded its indications to include painful osteoporotic and traumatic compression fractures, palliation of pathological fractures in combination with radiosurgery, and as an adjunct to neuraxis instrumentation. This chapter discusses PVP and percutaneous kyphoplasty (PVK) in the setting of vertebral metastatic disease.

Pathological osteolytic vertebral fractures resulting from tumor metastasis or myeloma are both relatively common as well as a significant source of painful morbidity. The skeletal system bears the brunt of neoplastic dissemination, occurring in 30 to 95% of the most common cancers including breast, prostate, lung, kidney, and thyroid. Among osseous structures, vertebrae are the most common site of spread and are the third most common site of metastases overall after the liver and lung.[1] Indeed, spinal metastases occur in approximately 40% of patients who die of cancer, and a staggering 5 to 10% of all cancer patients will have symptomatic spinal metastases at some point during their disease course.[1–3] The propensity for such high rates of vertebral involvement is likely due to the unique biology of the neuraxis and its relation to the most common primary cancer sites (including breast, prostate, and lung cancer). The vertebral and epidural hematogenous plexuses directly drain both breast and prostate tissue, and likely form a direct conduit with the pulmonary and genitourinary systems. Additionally, the axial skeleton contains the majority of red marrow in the human adult, and thus maintains a distinct cellular and extracellular milieu that may favor secondary tumor deposition and growth.[2]

Vertebral metastases occur throughout the neoplastic disease course, with events clustering around periods of primary tumor progression and with accelerating frequency during more advanced disease.[2] Both oncological disease burden and tumor histology play a significant prognostic role in patients with similar rates of axial skeleton disease burden. As would be expected from tumor-specific survival curves, primary lung tumors portend a significantly shorter survival than those of breast or prostate, a fact that must be taken into account when planning surgical interventions for vertebral pathological fractures. Furthermore, prognosis is typically improved with disease recurrence within the axial skeleton compared to visceral sites. For example, median survival is 24 months in women with metastatic breast cancer confined to the skeleton, whereas survival shrinks to 5 months with dual bone and liver disease.[2]

Although two thirds of all vertebral metastases are asymptomatic, the development of a pathological vertebral fracture significantly alters a patient's disease course and yields both increased morbidity and mortality. Saad et al[3] demonstrated this in an examination of a large group of patients with known malignant bone disease from multiple myeloma or other solid tissue tumors. Not only did they show a high rate of fracture for each tumor type in a 2-year period of observation (39% rate of fracture with breast cancer and 22% with other solid tumors), but also demonstrated that vertebral fracture was associated with a marked increase in mortality (up to 32% in patients with breast cancer compared with the nonfracture group). It is therefore critical to have a thorough understanding of the oncological disease burden when evaluating and informing patients on vertebral augmentation interventions.

The reasons for increased mortality after vertebral pathological fracture are likely multivariate, though the root causes are likely similar to those leading to elevated mortality after osteoporotic compression fractures. Tumor- and fracture-related pain is a key symptom leading to a cascade of morbid events, including impaired mobility, concomitant increased thromboembolic risk, progressive deformity with decreased pulmonary capacity and increased risk of cardiopulmonary collapse, deconditioning, loss of functional independence, social withdrawal, depression, increased narcotic analgesia intake, and associated mental status decline. Therapies designed to disrupt this cycle of decline can therefore have a profound impact on patient survival and quality of life even in the setting of metastatic disease. Vertebral augmentation with PVP and PVK in this patient population has increasingly demonstrated efficacy, technical feasibility, and low procedure morbidity. These minimally invasive procedures both involve percutaneous cannulation of the fractured vertebral body followed by injection of a liquid that polymerizes to a durable resin within the fractured body, thereby stabilizing the fracture. PVK entails the added step of insertion of a balloon tamp through the cannula followed by inflation, out-fracturing, and compaction of cancellous bone toward the cortical vertebral margin. The end plates are pushed apart, partially restoring vertebral body height

and focal kyphotic deformity. Polymer is then similarly injected into the cavity to harden and stabilize the fracture.

■ Patient Selection

As with any surgical procedure, proper patient evaluation and selection is critical to ensure a successful outcome. The assessment must include both medical and oncological status, and due diligence within both of these realms will guide the practitioner toward optimal diagnostic and treatment selection. Vertebral augmentation is an excellent option for patients who have severe systemic morbidity that precludes open surgical intervention, and it is likewise favored for healthy patients with osteolytic fractures that do not cause neurologic sequelae. Both of these groups, however, carry increased surgical risk from their concomitant cancer than that for the patient undergoing PVP or PVK for solely osteoporotic fracture.

Patients suitable for this procedure describe a typical axial or mechanical pain pattern that is aggravated with standing or twisting and relieved with lying flat. The location of the pain should correspond to the level of the fracture, an obvious but critically important point, as patients may have other vertebral levels with tumor involvement but no fracture. The biological pain of a tumor is differentiated from mechanical fracture pain by both constancy of pain throughout the day and night as well as its dull or throbbing qualities. This type of pain may be related to tumor release of local factors and cytokines, periosteal stretch, and local tissue production of endothelins and nerve growth factors.[1] Alternatively, neurologic pain should also be considered, as the compression or infiltration of a nerve root yields shooting pain in a dermatomal pattern and requires a decompressive procedure. An exception to this dictum is mechanical instability that causes activity-related impingement of the nerve root, where fracture stabilization prevents the intermittent nerve injury.

Eliciting a neurologic history and performing a thorough examination are important steps in the patient evaluation. Any neurologic symptoms, including paresis, sensory changes, bowel/bladder dysfunction, or changes in balance and ambulation, can indicate radicular or thecal sac compression by fracture or tumor. Changes in affect, cognition, speech, or cranial nerve dysfunction should be actively investigated due to the propensity for additional tumor–central nervous system (CNS) lesions. Patients should be counseled on the likely need for additional therapies for tumor control such as radiotherapy, as well as the need for optimization of systemic bone metabolism through pharmacological interventions to decrease future fractures. All the traditional risks of osteoporosis are present in this patient population, as well as the additional factors of cancer-related immobility, altered nutritional intake, and deranged osseous metabolism from tumor and treatment processes (chemotherapy or radiation). A detailed discussion of these pharmaceuticals is beyond the scope of this chapter. But it is important to note that bisphosphonates can reduce the incidence of additional-level fracture in both multiple myeloma and metastatic disease.[2,3] More recently, receptor activator of nuclear factor κ B (RANK) ligand inhibitors of osteoclast resorption have been approved for the prevention of skeleton-related events in patients with bone metastases from solid tumors such as breast and lung cancer and appear highly effective.[4]

Practitioners should attempt a reasonable trial of medical management for the mechanical fracture-related pain, and patients must understand that vertebral augmentation carries all the attendant risks of anesthesia and surgery. Active participation of other specialists adept at pain management should be sought, including anesthesia and palliative medicine, and conservative therapy should be considered, including local injections, systemic analgesia, and external orthosis. Preoperative laboratory investigations should confirm normal clotting (platelet level) and coagulation (international normalized ratio [INR]/prothrombin time [PT]/partial thromboplastin time [PTT]), as well as ensure where appropriate that there is no active or occult infection (*e.g.*, urinalysis with reflex culture). Bacteremia leading to hema-togenous seeding and infection of injected cement often requires a technically difficult corpectomy and attendant fusion, and can be easily avoided by maintaining a high index of suspicion. Antiplatelet agents should be temporarily discontinued.

Many patients with metastatic and myelomatous osseous disease suffer from hypercalcemia, most commonly seen in tumors of the lung, breast, and kidney and in myeloma and lymphoma. Tumor production of humoral and paracrine factors, including parathyroid hormone–related peptide, nurtures an osteolytic environment and deranged bone metabolism.[2] Early symptoms include fatigue, anorexia, and constipation, and can progress to renal and cardiovascular collapse. Patients therefore may suffer from the dual hit of metastatic vertebral fracture as well as a deranged metabolism leading to osteoporotic fracture.

Multimodal neuraxis imaging is a required step for preoperative planning to ensure a successful augmentation outcome. Complete magnetic resonance imaging (MRI) evaluation of the brain and spine should be a standard practice for patients with known CNS metastatic disease due to the propensity of multiple metastases. T2-weighted, fat-suppression, or short tau inversion recovery (STIR) sequences delineate the acuity of fracture, edema, and reparative activity. Bone scintigraphy can provide a further index of fracture-site metabolism, with increased activity correlating with a greater response to augmentation.[5] Both modalities can assist with symptomatic fracture localization when multiple fractures are present. Computed tomography (CT) scan provides valuable characterization of fracture morphology, vertebral height, pedicle width, trabecular disruption (characterized by intravertebral gas), and violation/retropulsion of the posterior cortical wall. We routinely obtain anteroposterior (AP) and lateral X-rays to facilitate accurate counting and to provide a corresponding view of the intraoperative fluoroscopic guidance images. Dynamic radiography with supine and upright films delivers valuable information on both the degree of kyphotic deformity as well as fracture mobility. Up to 44% of patients have a radiographically relevant change in vertebral height; patients whose vertebral height does not change are considered fixed.[6]

Relative and absolute contraindications to vertebral augmentation for metastatic disease are listed in the **Text Box.**

Contraindications to Vertebral Augmentation for Metastatic Disease

Absolute Contraindications
- Ongoing local or systemic infection
- Asymptomatic fractures or those improving on medical therapy
- Spinal canal compromise resulting in myelopathy from
  - Retropulsed bone fragment
  - Epidural tumor
- Uncorrectable coagulopathy or ongoing local or systemic infection

Relative Contraindications
- Severe vertebral body collapse (> 75% loss of height)
- Radiculopathy in excess of vertebral body axial mechanical pain.
  - Vertebroplasty can be considered in the setting of radicular pain that is due to fracture-related mechanical instability or as an adjunct prior to open surgical decompression.
- Asymptomatic cortical margin disruption or epidural tumor resulting in severe stenosis

(Adapted from McGraw JK, Cardella J, Barr JD, et al; Society of Interventional Radiology Standards of Practice Committee. Society of Interventional Radiology quality improvement guidelines for percutaneous vertebroplasty. J Vasc Interv Radiol 2003;14(9 Pt 2):S311–S315. Reproduced with permission.)

Absolute contraindications include patients with disease characteristics previously discussed, including local or systemic infection, spinal canal compromise from retropulsed bone fragment or epidural tumor with associated myelopathy, and uncorrectable coagulopathy. Relative contraindications are more fluid and some practitioners have demonstrated procedural safety and good outcomes in these patients.[7] As described before, intermittent radiculopathy associated with mechanical instability responds to cement stabilization, and pre- or periopera-tive augmentation can be used as an adjunct to open surgical decompression. Asymptomatic cortical margin disruption or epidural tumor resulting in severe stenosis should not be considered an absolute contraindication as long as meticulous injection technique is used.

Procedure

Methylmethacrylate (MMA) is a clear, resistant, durable, and relatively inert compound that polymerizes to a resin through an exothermic reaction. The synthetic polymer of MMA (poly-methylmethacrylate [PMMA]) is typically in powder form and is mixed with a radiopacifier (e.g., barium sulfate) and benzoyl peroxide initiator.[8] The foremost mechanism of action of PMMA vertebral augmentation is mechanical fracture stabilization, with unknown contributions of thermal and cytotoxic effects. Laboratory studies have investigated the contribution of thermal necrosis and sensory nerve thermoablation. Sensory nerves require sustained temperature elevation to > 45°C for injury to occur, though one must consider the convective heat transfer properties of adjacent vasculature and cerebrospinal fluid (CSF) as cooling mechanisms to the polymerizing resin. Temperature measurements of the injection cavity after vertebral injection do not show sustained temperature elevation to support a contribution of elevated temperature as a means toward pain control.

Vertebral augmentation may be performed with local anesthesia, monitored anesthesia care (MAC), or general anesthesia depending on preoperative surgical risk stratification. Patients are placed prone with chest and pelvic bolsters to augment pulmonary dynamics, decrease intra-abdominal pressure, and optimize kyphotic deformity correction. Biplanar fluoroscopy is an important aid for accurate pedicle localization and PMMA monitoring during injection. We orient the AP view to a slight oblique angle so that a "down the barrel" view of the pedicle is obtained. Local anesthetic injection, skin puncture incision, and additional local injection on the periosteum are performed. Pedicle cannulation by trocar is started in the upper-outer corner of the pedicle to facilitate a slightly caudal and medial trajectory that will enable PMMA injection in the center and contralateral vertebral body. A lateral, extrapedicular approach can also be used, particularly in the lumbar spine, enabling the needle to cross the midline. These maneuvers may help avoid the need for a contralateral approach. The more recent advent of curved needles has also decreased the need for two needles and a contralateral approach. After trocar insertion to a depth of approximately 20 mm the pedicle/body junction will be reached; crossing this border with lateral X-ray guidance confirms safe passage lateral to the canal and enables an exaggerated medial trajectory. We direct the trocar tip just shy of the ventral cortical border. A vertebral biopsy can be performed at this stage if there is any question regarding fracture etiology.

If a kyphoplasty is performed, the stylet is withdrawn, balloon tamps inserted, and balloon inflation performed under fluoroscopic and manometric guidance. The balloon compacts cancellous bone and pushes the end plates apart. Inflation end points include restoration of vertebral body height, balloon-tamp contact with a cortical vertebral wall, and tamp pressure 300 psi or maximum balloon volume. We prefer PMMA curing to a toothpaste viscosity before injection to avoid cement migration during injection. The injection is performed under continuous fluoroscopic guidance with gentle and controlled pressure, and is continued until the posterior one-third vertebral line is reached. Continued injection beyond this threshold risks cement escape and deposition around neural elements. The total volume of injected cement is less important than obtaining an equivalent injection volume across the midline to avoid a toggling effect.

■ Outcome Studies

Although two recent and somewhat controversial studies of vertebroplasty in the *New England Journal of Medicine* have questioned the value of vertebroplasty in osteoporotic patients, available evidence suggests that vertebroplasty is very useful in the setting of tumor.[9,10] The predominant literature for vertebral augmentation efficacy in vertebral body metastasis consists of retrospective cohort or case series, and is subject to the bias that accompanies these types of studies. One prospective trial has recently been published with encouraging outcomes supporting PVP and PVK in this patient population.[11] Typical outcome criteria include pain control, functional recovery measured by performance of activities of daily living (ADLs) and "out-of-bed" days, deformity correction, and procedure-related morbidity. There has not been a prospective trial directly comparing PVP with PVK for metastatic fracture, although subgroup analyses have pointed to equivalency for these outcome criteria.

The available retrospective series of vertebral augmentation in metastatic and myeloma fractures show robust efficacy for pain control and functional status up to 1 year after intervention.[12,13] Other symptoms that are associated with neoplastic disease, including anxiety, drowsiness, fatigue, and depression, may also improve after intervention.[14] Rates of symptomatic procedural complications were low.

A meta-analysis of available trials concluded that there is level II evidence supporting PVK in osteolytic metastatic and myeloma lesions.[15] Intervention was described as safe and effective for alleviation of pain and improvement in functional status and quality of life, and results were maintained for 2 years. Initial corrections in sagittal deformity were not maintained on long-term follow-up. This review was followed by the Cancer Patient Fracture Evaluation (CAFE) trial,[11] a prospective, randomized, unblinded, multicenter trial comparing PVK with medical management for patients who had cancer and concurrent osteolytic vertebral fractures. Primary and secondary outcome measures (back-specific functional status, Karnofsky Performance Scale (KPS), analgesia use, activity levels, and radiographic deformity correction) at 1 month were significantly improved with PVK over medical management. Many of the improved outcome measures were maintained at 1 year, and adverse events were equivalent between the two groups.

Vertebral augmentation through PMMA polymerization throughout the trabecular network of the fractured vertebral body likely achieves much of its therapeutic effect by mechanical stabilization of the deformed neuraxis. Not only does it provide rigidity to an unstable spinal segment, but it also may prevent further kyphotic deformity and progressive sagittal imbalance (**Fig. 8.1**). Many of the above trials incorporated longitudinal analysis of standing plain radiographs postprocedure, and though many noted early (1 month) improvements in vertebral body height, sagittal alignment, and focal kyphosis after PVP or PVK, these improvements gradually returned to baseline or were equivalent to controls 1 to 2 years later. Therefore, deformity correction does not ap-

pear to have as robust improvement as functional outcomes.[16]

Percutaneous kyphoplasty does have an advantage over PVP in postprocedural deformity correction in mobile fractures due to inflation of the bone tamps and spreading of the end plates, though patient positioning on the operating table achieves the majority of procedural correction. Proper chest and pelvic bolstering can achieve an average of 10-degree correction, whereas bone tamp inflation adds an additional 3 degrees; approximately 3 degrees are lost immediately on standing.[17] Therefore, PVK may be indicated over PVP if a greater kyphosis correction is warranted.

Despite the benefit afforded these minimally invasive interventions in the avoidance of open surgical fixation, they still have associated morbidity that must be considered before inter-

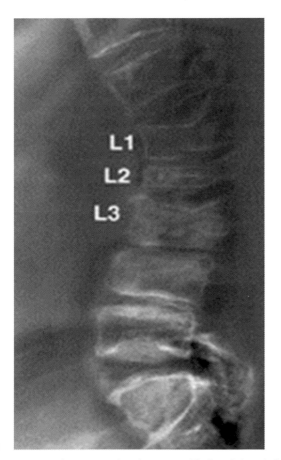

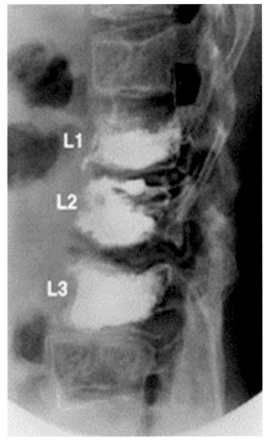

a   b

Fig. 8.1a,b Fracture height restored before **(a)** and after **(b)** vertebroplasty.

vention. Although the majority of adverse events are minor and asymptomatic, there is always the danger of a catastrophic outcome that requires that PVK/PVP be performed by experienced practitioners with access to facilities and expertise that can manage these rare events. The major complication rate, requiring corrective therapy or an unplanned increase in the level of care, or entailing permanent sequelae, rises from 1% (osteoporotic fracture) to 5% when there is neoplastic vertebral disease.[18]

Procedural complications include pedicle fracture and cement extravasation into adjacent soft tissue, disk, the venous system, neuroforamina, or spinal canal. Most extraosseous cement deposition is noted only by radiographs and is asymptomatic. Nevertheless, any extension of cement outside of the vertebral body into the spinal canal, neuroforamina, and anteriorly into vessels is an indication for procedure termination. Neuroforaminal impingement with radiculopathy can often be managed expectantly with adjuvant nonsteroidal anti-inflammatory drugs (NSAIDs) or steroids; continued radicular motor or sensory derangement should be surgically decompressed. Of course, any new evidence of postprocedural spinal cord injury requires emergent surgical exploration.

Cardiovascular complications from PMMA extravasation can range from minor hypotension to cardiopulmonary collapse after PMMA pulmonary embolism. Proposed mechanisms include direct injection into paravertebral veins causing local or distant vascular block, or through PMMA disruption of extracellular calcium mobilization and activation of coagulation pathways.[8] Careful technique including liberal use of fluoroscopy, termination of injection at the one-third posterior vertebral line, and cement injection only after polymerization to a viscous consistency all decrease the propensity for extravasation. PVK also has a lower extravasation risk than PVP, probably due to the balloon tamponade creating a bone "capsule" that can better contain cement as well as afford the use of a more viscous consistency.[19] However, PMMA interdigitation throughout the cancellous bone after PVP injection suggests a more robust stabilization than achieved with cavity injection after balloon tamponade. Overall, sys-

tematic review of PVP morbidity supports medical and neurologic complications up to 7% and 8%, respectively, whereas PVK has lower rates at 0.5% and 0%.[16]

Postprocedural fracture at a new level occurs in 7 to 20% of cases, though it is difficult to determine whether the fracture is related to local disruption of spinal dynamics or rather to new metastatic vertebral deposits and progression of osteoporosis. Retrospective analyses of fracture patterns show that the adjacent level constitutes approximately 40% of new fracture lesions, and that these adjacent fractures occur more often with pathological fractures and much sooner after vertebral augmentation (median 55 days compared with 127 days for distant fracture).[12,20] One can surmise that a treated segment acts as a pillar on adjacent levels, increasing stiffness of the segment and intervertebral joints, as well as increasing loads on adjacent segments.

■ Novel Uses and Future Applications

The minimally invasive character of PVP/PVK permits its use in combination with a number of treatment modalities for vertebral metastatic disease. Fracture stabilization with PMMA injected intraoperatively is an option in combination with open posterior decompression/fusion or with minimally invasive pedicle screw fixation, and may avoid the morbidity of open vertebrectomy and cage placement that may otherwise be required (**Fig. 8.2**). PVP can also be performed after multilevel reconstructive surgery to augment the anterior column, with vertebroplasty of the fractured vertebral body, adjacent vertebrae, or vertebrae with pedicle screws (**Fig. 8.3**).

Advancements in stereotactic spinal radiosurgery enable the delivery of a tumoricidal dose without injury to adjacent neural structures. Radiotherapy, however, likely increases fracture risk up to 40%, particularly with sclerotic lesions.[21] Vertebral augmentation should be considered as a neoadjuvant therapy for pathological fracture to prevent the relative

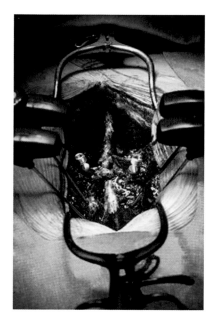

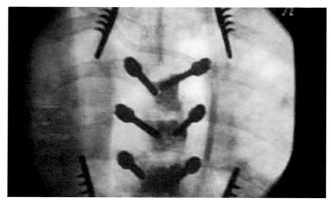

Fig. 8.2a,b A combination approach of open posterior fixation with vertebral body polymethylmethacrylate (PMMA) augmentation. **(a)** Intraoperative photograph demonstrating pedicle cannulation for cement injection. **(b)** Postoperative anteroposterior (AP) radiograph.

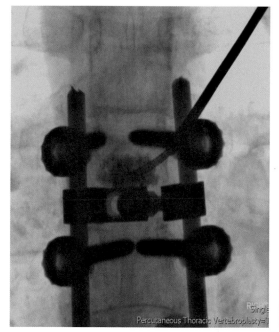

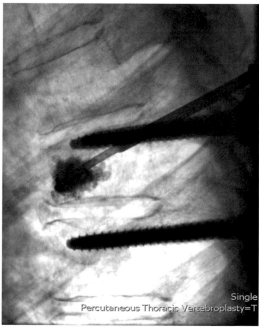

Fig. 8.3a,b Vertebroplasty after open posterior fixation in a patient with melanoma to prevent further collapse of the superior vertebral body of the construct. Anteroposterior **(a)** and lateral **(b)** views demonstrate the needle introduced using a lateral approach, coursing under the pedicle screw, and with the use of a curved needle to fill the anterior vertebral body.

likelihood of fracture progression after radiotherapy. A retrospective review did not find any negative interaction between radiation efficacy before and after vertebral augmentation.[22]

■ Chapter Summary

Vertebral compression fractures that are a result of metastatic disease and multiple myeloma are a source of significant suffering for patients, and fracture progression poses a risk for debilitating mechanical and neurologic spinal instability. Concurrently, many patients are high-risk candidates for open surgical stabilization due to neoplastic disease and its systemic treatment toxicity. PVP and PVK offer an effective minimally invasive option for fracture stabilization and symptom relief. Treatment efficacy has been demonstrated in retrospective case series and a limited number of prospective trials, and further investigation will help define patient selection and expected outcomes.

The spine is a common location for neoplastic dissemination, and up to 10% of cancer patients will suffer from symptomatic pathological vertebral fractures from metastases during the course of disease. Such fractures carry a significant morbidity, including debilitating pain, progressive deformity, and the risk of neurologic decline. Conservative treatment options, excluding external orthosis and narcotic pain control, are often ineffective and can be difficult to manage, whereas open surgical stabilization is a high-risk venture for patients suffering from systemic disease and toxic treatments.

Percutaneous vertebroplasty and kyphoplasty are minimally invasive vertebral stabilization options that have shown efficacy in this vulnerable patient population. The procedure involves cannulation into the fractured vertebral body followed by injection of PMMA, which will exothermically polymerize to a rigid resin. Kyphoplasty entails the added step of balloon tamp inflation within the vertebral body to increase vertebral height before cement stabilization. The two procedures are relatively easy to execute and are typically performed on an outpatient basis. Available evidence suggests strong efficacy in the relief of fracture pain, increased patient function, decreased use of narcotics, and stabilization if not correction of focal kyphotic deformity.

Careful patient selection, including those with axial mechanical back pain without neurologic sequelae, as well as preoperative planning with appropriate imaging sequences, increases treatment success and reduces potential morbidity. Vertebral augmentation is a relatively safe procedure, though there is the potential for rare catastrophic neurologic or cardiopulmonary events, and thus careful and diligent technique is vital. PVP and PVK are excellent minimally invasive treatment options for fracture stabilization, and can be used in combination with tumoricidal therapies for local disease control.

Pearls

◆ Forty percent of cancer patients will have vertebral metastatic disease, of which 10% will be symptomatic.
◆ Vertebral augmentation is a minimally invasive technique that decreases vertebral fracture pain and increases functional outcomes, likely through mechanical stabilization of the spine.
◆ Perioperative patient positioning can correct focal kyphotic deformity by 10 degrees.
◆ PVP/PVK can be used in conjunction with tumoricidal therapy (i.e., radiation) for local disease control.

Pitfalls

◆ Preoperative evidence of focal spinal cord dysfunction from fracture or tumor is an absolute contraindication to vertebral augmentation.
◆ Terminate PMMA injection if there is any evidence of cement extravasation posteriorly into the spinal canal or neuroforamen or anteriorly into a vascular structure or after reaching the posterior one-third vertebral line.
◆ PMMA injection volume does not correlate with symptom relief; therefore, avoid overinjection of polymer.

References

Five Must-Read References

1. Mercadante S. Malignant bone pain: pathophysiology and treatment. Pain 1997;69:1–18

2. Coleman RE. Clinical features of metastatic bone disease and risk of skeletal morbidity. Clin Cancer Res 2006;12(20 Pt 2):6243s–6249s

3. Saad F, Lipton A, Cook R, Chen YM, Smith M, Coleman R. Pathologic fractures correlate with reduced survival in patients with malignant bone disease. Cancer 2007;110:1860–1867

4. Henry DH, Costa L, Goldwasser F, et al. Randomized, double-blind study of denosumab versus zoledronic acid in the treatment of bone metastases in patients with advanced cancer (excluding breast and prostate cancer) or multiple myeloma. J Clin Oncol 2011;29:1125–1132

5. Maynard AS, Jensen ME, Schweickert PA, Marx WF, Short JG, Kallmes DF. Value of bone scan imaging in predicting pain relief from percutaneous vertebroplasty in osteoporotic vertebral fractures. AJNR Am J Neuroradiol 2000;21:1807–1812

6. Faciszewski T, McKiernan F. Calling all vertebral fractures classification of vertebral compression fractures: a consensus for comparison of treatment and outcome. J Bone Miner Res 2002;17:185–191

7. Hentschel SJ, Burton AW, Fourney DR, Rhines LD, Mendel E. Percutaneous vertebroplasty and kyphoplasty performed at a cancer center: refuting proposed contraindications. J Neurosurg Spine 2005;2:436–440

8. Leggat PA, Smith DR, Kedjarune U. Surgical applications of methyl methacrylate: a review of toxicity. Arch Environ Occup Health 2009;64:207–212

9. Kallmes DF, Comstock BA, Heagerty PJ, et al. A Randomized Trial of Vertebroplasty for Osteoporotic Spinal Fractures. N Engl J Med 2009;361:569–579

10. Buchbinder R, Osborne RH, Ebeling PR, et al. A Randomized Trial of Vertebroplasty for Painful Osteoporotic Vertebral Fractures. N Engl J Med 2009;361:557–568

11. Berenson J, Pflugmacher R, Jarzem P, et al; Cancer Patient Fracture Evaluation (CAFE) Investigators. Balloon kyphoplasty versus non-surgical fracture management for treatment of painful vertebral body compression fractures in patients with cancer: a multicentre, randomised controlled trial. Lancet Oncol 2011;12:225–235

12. Burton AW, Mendoza T, Gebhardt R, et al. Vertebral compression fracture treatment with vertebroplasty and kyphoplasty: experience in 407 patients with 1,156 fractures in a tertiary cancer center. Pain Med 2011;12:1750–1757

13. Jha RM, Hirsch AE, Yoo AJ, Ozonoff A, Growney M, Hirsch JA. Palliation of compression fractures in cancer patients by vertebral augmentation: a retrospective analysis. J Neurointerv Surg 2010;2:221–228

14. Mendoza TR, Koyyalagunta D, Burton AW, et al. Changes in pain and other symptoms in patients with painful multiple myeloma-related vertebral fracture treated with kyphoplasty or vertebroplasty. J Pain 2012;13:564–570

15. Bouza C, López-Cuadrado T, Cediel P, Saz-Parkinson Z, Amate JM. Balloon kyphoplasty in malignant spinal fractures: a systematic review and meta-analysis. BMC Palliat Care 2009;8:12

16. Mendel E, Bourekas E, Gerszten P, Golan JD. Percutaneous techniques in the treatment of spine tumors: what are the diagnostic and therapeutic indications and outcomes? Spine 2009;34(22, Suppl):S93–S100

17. Voggenreiter G. Balloon kyphoplasty is effective in deformity correction of osteoporotic vertebral compression fractures. Spine 2005;30:2806–2812

18. McGraw JK, Cardella J, Barr JD, et al; Society of Interventional Radiology Standards of Practice Committee. Society of Interventional Radiology quality improvement guidelines for percutaneous vertebroplasty. J Vasc Interv Radiol 2003;14(9 Pt 2):S311–S315

19. Barragán-Campos HM, Vallée JN, Lo D, et al. Percutaneous vertebroplasty for spinal metastases: complications. Radiology 2006;238:354–362

20. Trout AT, Kallmes DF, Kaufmann TJ. New fractures after vertebroplasty: adjacent fractures occur significantly sooner. AJNR Am J Neuroradiol 2006;27:217–223

21. Rose PS, Laufer I, Boland PJ, et al. Risk of fracture after single fraction image-guided intensity-modulated radiation therapy to spinal metastases. J Clin Oncol 2009;27):5075–5079

22. Hirsch AE, Jha RM, Yoo AJ, et al. The use of vertebral augmentation and external beam radiation therapy in the multimodal management of malignant vertebral compression fractures. Pain Physician 2011;14:447–458

9

Surgical Complications and Their Avoidance

Michelle J. Clarke

■ Introduction

Operative treatment of metastatic spine disease is palliative and targeted to improve health-related quality of life (HRQOL). Surgical treatment is usually reserved for patients with metastatic spinal cord compression or spinal instability. The primary goals of surgery are to decompress neurologic elements to prevent, stabilize, or improve neurologic deficit, provide a safe margin for radiotherapy, stabilize the spinal column, and achieve local disease control. Despite these relatively clear indications, surgeons must not lose sight of the bigger picture: although palliative spine surgery can improve HRQOL,[1] complications will lengthen the hospitalization[2] and negatively impact the quality of life. Additionally, surgical complications may delay or prevent adjuvant radiation and chemotherapy for the patient's primary disease. This chapter discusses specific complications and their avoidance.

■ Patient Selection

For surgical treatment of metastatic spine disease to be successful, a patient must be able to make a meaningful recovery. Accurately assessing the extent of disease and the medical risks of the procedure are important for prognostication and surgical decision making. In

most cases, surgery is considered semi-urgent and a thorough but expedited workup is appropriate. Even in emergent cases of catastrophic neurologic deterioration, medical and oncological consultation should be obtained.

Surgical intervention in metastatic spine disease is intended to protect or restore neurologic function; thus, a surgical candidate must meet functional criteria to be considered for surgery. Poor performance status may be a contraindication for surgery. Exceptions to this include patients with pathological fractures that have a poor performance status due to pain-related immobility, or patients with rapid neurologic deterioration in the previous 24 to 48 hours.

Although they have been refined, the original Patchell criteria are an appropriate starting point. Patients should have a life expectancy of at least 3 months but preferably 6 months to achieve a measurably enhanced quality of life following the procedure,[1] although this may be shortening with the advent of percutaneous and other minimally invasive procedures. Widely metastatic disease may be a contraindication for surgery. Thus, oncological workup may include needle biopsy of the spine or other accessible lesion to obtain pathological diagnosis of the primary tumor. Metastatic workup including chest, abdomen, and pelvis computed tomography (CT); bone scan; pan-spine magnetic resonance imaging (MRI) and brain MRI; and positron emission tomography can be considered to determine the extent of disease. Radiation-responsive tumors require particular thoughtfulness related to stability and the cause of neurology. A patient may be better served without a surgical procedure; however, cord compression involving bone fragments due to a pathological burst fracture may still require operative intervention, even in a radiosensitive tumor.

The surgical procedure must be well planned. In some cases, the burden of disease in the spinal column makes surgical resection or reconstruction technically impossible. The surgeon must be able to achieve a worthwhile decompression and restore biomechanical stability to the spinal column. If either of these goals cannot be met, the patient may not be a surgical candidate.

If a patient is deemed an oncological and functional candidate for surgery, a patient must be able to tolerate the anticipated procedure. For a standard extracavitary approach, vertebrectomy, and stabilization, it is reasonable to estimate a 2-L blood loss and a 6-hour operative time, with the patient in the prone position. These estimates may enable the medical and anesthesia physicians to determine the surgical risk. Patients without a high probability of surviving the procedure should not undergo it, even in the face of imminent paralysis.

Appropriate patient selection and anticipation of adverse events based on comorbid medical conditions is the most important component of complication avoidance. Detailed discussion of appropriate patient surgical selection is discussed in Chapter 1.

Preoperative Evaluation and Preparation

Once it has been determined that a patient is a candidate for surgery, a thoughtful approach should be employed, even in urgent or emergent cases, to minimize oncology-specific risk factors. In most cases, the surgical target has been chosen because of potential or actual neurologic decline due to compression of instability or pain related to instability. The tumor at the surgical target itself may warrant preoperative intervention to decrease the surgical risk as discussed in the embolization section below. Additionally, the overall disease burden and the effect of previous radiation or chemotherapy that the patient may have already have undergone can greatly affect surgical outcome. Thus, this section discusses the hematologic and neurotoxic considerations that should be carefully addressed in the preoperative period.

Hemorrhage

Although sudden catastrophic hemorrhage is rare in metastatic spine tumor surgery, a number of factors lead to high blood loss. Thus, surgical planning should include strategies to correct hematologic abnormalities, minimize blood loss, and manage intraoperative hemorrhage.[3]

Coagulation Abnormalities

The oncology patient's natural hemostatic response may be disrupted by the primary disease, especially in cases of hematologic malignancies, those involving the liver, or following certain nonsurgical therapies resulting in bone marrow suppression. Preoperatively, a complete coagulation panel is imperative, with factor correction as necessary. Additionally, large-bore intravenous access or central lines should be considered preoperatively. Fluid and blood can be infused through warmers, which in conjunction with body warmers may reduce intraoperative coagulopathies. Unfortunately, due to the risk of metastasizing tumor from the surgical site, blood salvage equipment should not be used.

Intraoperatively, attention should be paid to nontumoral blood loss and tumoral bleeding. In addition to standard soft tissue and bony bleeding, epidural venous bleeding can be extensive. Patient positioning can minimize intraabdominal pressure, and the use of multiple hemostatic agents is helpful. Postoperatively, hematologic parameters should be monitored, as fluid shifts and blood loss via drains may be significant.

Conversely, cancer patients are often hypercoagulable, leading to disseminated intravascular coagulation, deep venous thromboses (DVTs), and pulmonary emboli (PEs). Intraoperatively, sequential compression devices (SCDs) are used during these often long procedures with the patient in the prone position. Postoperatively, consideration should be given to early mobilization, the continued use of SCDs, and the use of anticoagulants such as subcutaneous heparin. This is especially important in patients who have suffered neurologic deterioration and recent loss of mobility. A low threshold for lower extremity Doppler ultrasound to investigate possible DVTs and aggressive treatment with intravascular filter placement and anticoagulation are indicated. Similarly, surgeons should have a low threshold for investigation of suspected PEs and should aggressively treat them upon diagnosis.

Preoperative Embolization

Tumors, especially vascular lesions, are often difficult to cauterize and do not stop bleeding until they are completely resected. Certain lesions may benefit from preoperative embolization to decrease intraoperative hemorrhage, not only to reduce the physiological stress on the patient by decreasing blood loss,[4] but also to make it easier for the surgeon to visualize and complete the procedure efficiently and safely. Specifically, renal cell carcinoma, follicular thyroid carcinoma, neuroendocrine tumors, and tumors of unknown histology with suggestions of hypervascularity on imaging studies should be considered for embolization.[3] In other cases, if a vascular lesion is suspected and embolization is not possible, en bloc resection can be attempted to avoid violating the tumor (discussed in Chapter 4). An additional advantage to embolization is the ability to localize major spinal segmental feeding arteries such as the artery of Adamkiewicz. Rhizotomy or nerve root sacrifice at this level can lead to anterior spinal artery ischemia and spinal cord infarction and should be avoided if possible.

Operative Positioning

Protection of both the central and peripheral nervous systems is imperative in metastatic spine tumor patients. Most patients are selected for surgical intervention due to spinal cord compression or instability resulting in neurologic compromise. Thus, care must be taken not to worsen spinal cord compression during positioning. Documenting a preoperative examination, obtaining preoperative electrophysiological monitoring baselines, and performing awake or fiberoptic intubation in cervical cases should be considered. Careful positioning, including log-roll or Jackson table sandwich techniques and pinions are especially important to protect the spinal cord. Postposition electrophysiological monitoring and wake-up tests to assess neurologic status and pre-draping imaging studies to assess preopeative alignment are helpful. Should any study demonstrate decreased neurologic function, the surgeon must consider reversing the positioning, waking the patient, and employing a set spinal cord injury protocol as discussed below (see Neurologic Injury).

Oncology patients also require special attention to their peripheral nervous system. Many patients have been exposed to neurotoxic chemotherapeutic agents prior to undergoing surgical intervention. These agents may increase their risk of position-dependent injuries such as ulnar neuropathies; thus, special attention should be paid to table padding and straps. Finally, the operating room staff should note and protect any chemotherapeutic ports the patient may have in place for systemic treatment.

◼ Intraoperative Complications: Prevention and Minimization

The basic tenets of spine surgery are the key to a successful procedure in the oncology patient. Even in emergent situations, the surgeon must thoroughly understand the regional anatomy, obtain adequate exposure, and employ gentle tissue handling techniques. Most importantly, pathological changes in anatomy must be understood and regional structures of vital importance must be identified before proceeding. It is wise to work from normal to pathological anatomy to maintain orientation. Tumors are notoriously unpredictable in their behavior: ensuring that all structures are well visualized and protected in a systematic fashion allows a surgeon to react confidently in the face of unexpected complications such as sudden hemorrhage. Finally, respecting natural tissue planes, maintaining reasonable hemostasis, and ensuring that soft tissue remains vital and perfused will lessen the physiological stress of surgery and improve healing in patients who may be weakened by their primary disease and treatments. A thoughtful and deliberate approach to these technically challenging surgeries and complex patients will improve the chance of success.

Neurologic Injury

One of the major goals of spine surgery for metastasis is the prevention or potential reversal of neurologic deficit due to spinal cord compression. However, one of the most feared surgical complications is spinal cord injury. Preoperative, intraoperative, and postoperative practices may reduce the risk of neurologic deterioration. Additionally, appropriate intraoperative and postoperative response to suspected spinal cord injury may minimize or reverse potential deficits.

Preoperatively, unless medically contraindicated, patients with new neurologic deficit who are undergoing preoperative medical and oncological workup should receive high-dose steroids to decrease spinal cord edema.[5] Commonly, this takes the form of a loading dose and subsequent maintenance doses. The standard is now 10 mg of dexamethasone bolus and 4 to 6 mg every 6 hours is a reasonable starting point, although this standard remains controversial. Ultimately, following surgery, the drug is tapered down to oncologically useful doses.

Intraoperatively, for cases involving spinal cord decompression, we commonly use somatosensory evoked potential (SSEP) and motor evoked potential (MEP) monitoring, and freerunning electromyogram (EMG) can be used in cases of root compression. Prepositioning neurophysiological baselines should be obtained and maintained throughout the procedure. If signals are poor, consideration can be given to a postpositioning wake-up test. The surgical, anesthesia, and neuromonitoring teams should be well versed in their response to a decreased monitoring response.[6] The surgical team should consider whether new or increased mechanical cord compression has occurred, such as hematoma, instrumentation malposition, or deformity correction, and consider decompressing or reversing it if possible. The anesthesia team should ensure that the patient is normothermic and hemodynamically resuscitated, and that there were no changes to anesthetic/medication delivery, and should consider raising mean arterial pressure to 90 mm Hg. The monitoring team should check its equipment and leads to ensure there is no technical problem with the device. Steroid bolus can be considered if not already given.

Postoperatively, at the discretion of the surgical team, blood pressure may be artificially elevated and steroids continued in an effort to increase cord perfusion and decrease edema. This is especially helpful in patients with new deficits, or in instances where it is suspected that the vascular perfusion pattern of the spinal cord is altered, such as multiple nerve root and radicular artery sacrifices.

Adjacent Organ Injury

Epidural tumor surgery may be complicated by injury to an adjacent structure. Surgical planning to minimize such transgressions includes understanding anatomy distortion through pathological processes, protecting adjacent structures (for example, placing ureteral stents or employing preoperative endovascular vessel sacrifice), and minimizing multiple-compartment surgeries (for instance, using an extracavitary approach to thoracic spinal lesions while avoiding the chest cavity). A plan for intraoperative iatrogenic adjacent organ injury should be considered preoperatively.

Spinal Fluid Leak

Cerebrospinal fluid (CSF) extravagation may complicate wound healing and result in intradural tumor seeding (**Fig. 9.1**). Although best

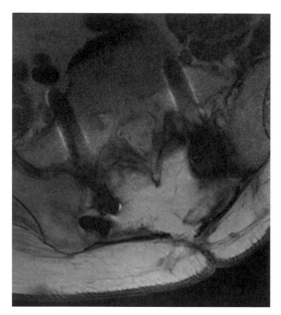

Fig. 9.1 Patient with inadequately repaired primary dural tear and improperly closed fascia who has developed a pseudomeningocele immediately prior to his first wound dehiscence. The patient required three surgical revisions including vascularized rotational flap, resulting in 4-month hospitalization. Two years later he has a palpable but stable pseudomeningocele and continued low-pressure headaches.

avoided, if dural tears occur in oncological cases, they should be aggressively treated in a similar fashion to those occurring in other spine surgeries.[7] Dural rents should be repaired primarily or using a patch graft if the rent is too large for primary closure. Similarly, if rhizotomy is performed, the root should be tied or clipped securely to prevent CSF egress. Oversewing a muscle pledget or using a dural sealant can be considered. When a durotomy is irreparable, the use of a lumbar drain for several days will decrease the hydrostatic pressure on the repair. Additionally, CSF absorption may be compromised in irradiated tissue, thus even low-volume leaks are prone to wound healing problems.[3]

Probably the most important principle in treating a CSF leak is adequate soft tissue coverage around the dura. CSF leaks are unlikely to heal if there is dead space around the dura, a situation not uncommon after surgery for spine metastases. Surgeons should have a very low threshold for involving their plastic surgery colleagues to provide healthy tissue coverage in the setting of a CSF leak.

The CSF leaks become very difficult to treat when the operative cavity is open to the pleural space such as a transthoracic approach or a costotransversectomy with pleural violation. In these cases, exquisite attention must be paid to closing the dura and potentially separating the area of leak from the negative pressure chest cavity and chest tube. Patients with mental status decline and suspected CSF leak, especially those with nearby negative pressure suction devices, should have an urgent CT to rule out remote hemorrhages. In both of these cases, suction should be immediately stopped, the CSF leak located and repaired, and life-threatening hemorrhages treated to avoid potentially fatal brain herniation. Of note, in multispecialty cases involving CSF leak, attention should be paid to drains to gravity and chest tubes left by other surgical services; chest tubes to water-seal and drains to gravity, which must be clearly communicated if a non–spine service is closing the incision.

Although a stable subfascial pseudomeningocele is an acceptable result, any transcutaneous CSF fistula must be promptly addressed to promote wound healing and prevent infection and meningitis. Unfortunately, as with other wound issues, CSF leaks, especially transcutaneous fistulas, will delay adjuvant therapy. Patients should not be treated with local radiation or systemic chemotherapy until the wound is completely healed. Aggressive treatment including early reoperation, detailed attempts at primary repair, and adequate soft tissue coverage are indicated. In cases of transcutaneous CSF leak, a subfascial wound drain can be placed as a last resort to provide CSF with a distant egress to promote wound healing, but avoiding suction to prevent a negative pressure scenario will decrease the risk of the leak's worsening, overdrainage, and other adverse events such as subdural hematoma or pneumocephalus creation. Other CSF diversion tactics including lumbar drainage, lumbo- or ventriculoperitoneal shunts, and plastic surgery closure may be required to heal the primary wound in challenging cases.

Vascular Injury

Anatomic distortion due to pathological anatomy makes vascular transgression a risk. Preoperative angiography, temporary balloon occlusion, and permanent vessel sacrifice may be useful preoperative adjuncts, especially in lesions encasing the vertebral arteries of the cervical spine. Promptly alerting the anesthesia team to potential high-volume blood loss and obtaining immediate assistance from the vascular surgery or interventional department may be required.

Esophageal/Bowel Injury

Proximity to the spine, pathological distortion by tumoral processes, and radiation-related scarring may result in violation of the gastrointestinal tract. Prompt attention from a general surgeon or otolaryngologist may be needed for primary repair or diversion procedures. Additionally, alterations in the antibiotic regimen and nutritional parameters should be addressed. Unfortunately, spillage of gastrointestinal contents greatly increases the risk of infection, especially complicating cases involving instrumentation.

Chyle Leak

Chyle leaks may occur during transthoracic procedures and are often difficult to detect. Milky fluid in the operative cavity may be noted, but the problem may not become apparent until the postoperative period. In this case, assistance from the thoracic surgery service may be required, and diet alterations have proved to be the best therapy.

■ Postoperative Complications

Instability and Pseudarthrosis

Attention should be paid to stabilizing and reconstructing the spinal column to promote pain control and early mobilization. In some pa-tients, stabilization alone to reduce the pain of pathological fracture may be the indicated treatment. In other patients, a 360-degree spinal canal decompression will result in the elimination of a large portion of the stabilizing components of the spinal column, thus requiring extensive reconstruction. Typically, subaxial decompression involves resection of a vertebral body and anterior canal tumor requiring stabilization; however, the occipitocervical junction is often best approached via posterior decompression and fusion alone. See Chapter 6 for a thorough discussion of fixation/fusion and Chapter 8 for vertebroplasty/kyphoplasty indications and techniques.

In general, instrumentation designed for degenerative, deformity, and trauma surgery is employed, although specific guidelines for instrumentation choice and construct design in tumor patients should be considered. In all cases, the initiation of cytotoxic adjuvant therapies, high metabolic demands of the cancer and cancer treatments, and the common use of steroids make fusion difficult to achieve. Thus, surgeons should consider this a stabilization procedure as opposed to a true arthrodesis and fusion. Ongoing tumor surveillance and radiotherapy planning using MRI means that surgeons should attempt to reduce the amount of metal artifact by judicious use of crosslinks or alternating screws. Polyetheretherketone (PEEK), polymethylmethacrylate (PMMA), and allograft or autograft bone struts may be preferable to titanium cages due to their large amount of metal artifact, although expandable metal cages offer safety and simplicity. Newer cobalt Chromalloy rods and screw heads may lead to increased imaging artifact, and should be avoided if possible.

Bone quality can affect the surgical plan, and therefore contingency plans must be in place before the operation has started. Bone weakened by osteoporosis or previous radiotherapy may be difficult to instrument. It may be wise to increase load-sharing by increasing the number of levels fixated, or increase pullout strength by augmenting vertebral bodies with the addition of PMMA or large-diameter screws. Generally in these patients it is recommended to err on the side of overfixation.

Late instrumentation complications are particularly challenging (**Fig. 9.2**). Following treatment, loose instrumentation or pathological fracture may require attention. Unfortunately, reoperation often reveals porcelain-white bone and gray surrounding tissue. Upsizing the instrumentation to obtain a mechanical fixation is important, but the surgeon may want to consider extending the construct to an area of greater viability, outside of the radiation field, for example. Often the best solution is to forgo further surgery; only symptomatic patients should be operated on, and with the awareness that wound and bone healing may become a major problem.

Infection and Wound

Surgical-site infection or wound dehiscence is a very serious complication. Not only will additional interventions and suffering occur, but patients will be unable to undergo local radiation or systemic chemotherapies until wound healing is complete, which can directly affect survival. Wound complications have been reported in up to a third of patients undergoing surgical treatment of spinal neoplasms.[8] Cancer patients are particularly susceptible to infection due to the primary disease, malnutrition, tissue damage due to recent radiation, immunosuppression due to chemotherapeutic agents, and immunosuppression related to administration of steroids that often occurs in the setting of metastatic spinal cord compression.[9,10] It is ideal to delay surgical treatment until an oncological treatment window is beneficial. However, most cases are treated emergently due to neurologic compromise. Despite the increased risk of infection, high-dose corticosteroids should still be administered as a neuroprotectant in patients suffering from symptomatic high-grade spinal cord compression. Although many of these risk factors are unmodifiable, filgrastim (Neupogen) may be used to recover the absolute neutrophil count in severely neutropenic patients.[3] Additionally, a dietary consult may be beneficial, as many patients are malnourished due to their primary disease process, which will impair healing.

Perioperative antibiotics should be administered prior to surgical incision and continued postoperatively. Routinely, antibiotics such as cefazolin, vancomycin, or both, are used to cover skin flora. Ampicillin/gentamycin my be added of operating through the abdominal cavity, or ciprofloxacin/flagyl if an oropharyngeal approach is required. Antibiotics should be redosed appropriately throughout the procedure and continued for 24 hours postoperatively or while drains are in place. Although it is not standard, topical vancomycin powder may be applied in the wound as an additional precaution.

Prior to final closure, the wound is thoroughly irrigated with saline. The wound is approximated in tight layers and prophylactic soft tissue closure can be considered at the index procedure.[8] A suture that has a longer absorption time course or even a permanent suture may be useful due to the slow wound healing in oncological patients. Subfascial drains are used to minimize dead space, prevent the accumulation of fluid that can act as an infective nidus, and eliminate transdermal wound drainage. The wound is kept covered for 24 hours until the epithelium is sealed. In patients with prior radiation, sutures are left in place for a longer period than standard.

Adjustment in adjuvant therapy scheduling is usually required to promote wound healing. Conformal treatment such as intensity-modulated radiation therapy (IMRT) has lessened the risk of wound breakdown associated with external beam radiotherapy; however, optimal radiation–surgery/surgery–radiation timing guidelines remain elusive.[11] Normally, a 3-week postoperative healing period prior to resumption of chemotherapy or local radiation therapy is preferred.

Patients and their families are given strict instructions to watch the wound for signs of infection or wound breakdown and to bring the patient for examination as soon as possible if it occurs. Of note, immunosuppressed patients may not mount a strong immune response; thus, late infections or serious infections, despite an absence of purulence and laboratory markers, should be considered a possibility. Baseline

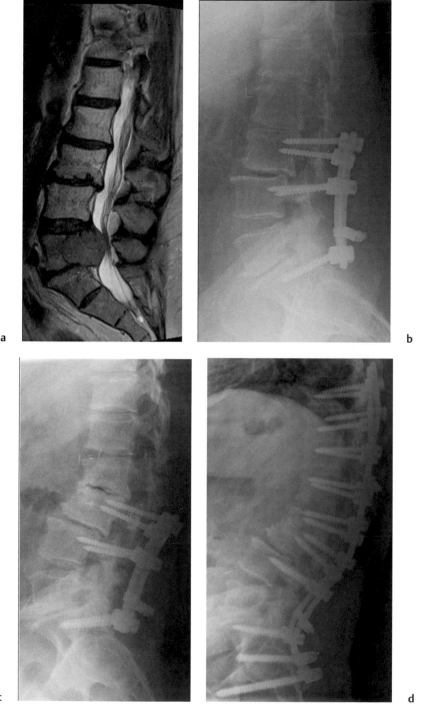

Fig. 9.2a–d A patient with a renal cell carcinoma metastasis to L5 **(a)** underwent resection and stabilization from a posterior approach **(b)** followed by radiation. Although the patient demonstrated instrumentation loosening and lack of bony fusion, he was asymptomatic until 3 years postoperatively, when he developed a painful adjacent segment compression fracture **(c)**. This was biopsy negative and the patient was treated with T10 to pelvis stabilization **(d),** with evidence of bony fusion in the nonradiated bed 2 years postoperatively.

infectious lab tests, cultures, and imaging should be obtained. Early washout, wound revision, and intravenous antibiotics must be considered and can be tailored based on susceptibilities. To resume adjuvant therapy as expeditiously as possible, it is preferable to close the wound primarily or use flaps during initial washout as opposed to multiple washouts or leaving the wound packed open.[12]

Wound dehiscence and poor healing are common in metastatic tumor patients even without a primary surgical site infection. In patients who have undergone preoperative radiation at the surgical site, the surgeon should take pains to debride unhealthy tissue prior to closure. Should regional tissue be unviable at the index procedure, or if this becomes apparent by a postoperative wound dehiscence, vascularized flaps may be required for closure. A plastic surgeon should be consulted for consideration of rotational or free flaps. It is important to culture superficial and deep tissue in the setting of wound dehiscence, as patients may harbor an infection without mounting an obvious response.

■ Follow-Up

Following surgical treatment, multidisciplinary coordination is required to ensure appropriate follow-up and adjuvant treatment. Normally, patients return for a wound examination or send a digital picture of their incision 2 to 3 weeks postoperatively, prior to embarking on further local or systemic treatment, to ensure that the wound has fully epithelialized and is without signs of breakdown. It is important to follow instrumented patients at regular intervals to ensure that there are no new pathological fractures or instrumentation issues.

Oncologically, the patient should be monitored and treated in conjunction with medical and radiation oncology. Although monitoring intervals usually range from 3 to 6 months, they vary based on tumor histology and treatment planning. Any recurrence of pain or neurologic decline prompts swift reimaging. In one series

of surgically treated spine metastases of mixed pathology, recurrence rates were as high as 60% at 6 months and 70% at 1 year.[13] Although MRI usually provides adequate information, instrumentation artifact may necessitate a CT myelogram to definitively diagnose cord compression. If a surgical lesion is noted, once again, based on overall patient health, functional status, and disease burden, further surgeries may be warranted and may prolong survival.[14]

■ Chapter Summary

Surgical treatment of metastatic spine disease is important to improve patient quality of life. However, surgical complications may have dire consequences for overall survival as they may preclude further life-prolonging adjuvant therapies. A methodical approach and meticulous attention to detail are required for optimal results. Appropriate patient selection is essential to achieve a good outcome; patients must be able to tolerate the anticipated surgery with the hope of regaining or maintaining a good quality of life for a reasonable period of time to make the intervention worthwhile. Patients should be medically optimized and coagulation factors normalized prior to surgery. A thoughtful approach, including preoperative embolization, attention to positioning, and the use of intraoperative electrophysiological monitoring, should be considered. Surgeons should take care to optimize wound healing, as this is the most common and often most difficult complication and delays adjuvant therapy. This includes definitive repair of CSF leaks and the use of lumbar drains, copious wound irrigation, and a multilayered closure to eliminate dead space. Patients should have close follow-up in the perioperative period by a multidisciplinary team.

Pearls

◆ Expected survival from primary disease, medical clearance for surgery, and functional status are vital for appropriate prognostication and suitability for surgery (see Chapter 1).

- Medically optimize the patient prior to surgery, including normalization of coagulation factors.
- Completely understand the local anatomy, and work from normal to pathological to maintain orientation.
- Embolize suspected vascular tumors preoperatively.
- Protect the neural elements throughout the procedure, acting promptly and with forethought if there is a decline in neurophysiological monitoring.
- Perioperative antibiotics and impeccable closure are required.
- Intervene early and aggressively in any suspected wound infection or dehiscence.
- Local radiation and systemic chemotherapy should be withheld until the wound is healed.

- Multidisciplinary follow-up and adjuvant treatment planning are essential.

Pitfalls

- Inadequate recognition of the pathological distortion of normal anatomy can result in catastrophic complications.
- Inattention to closure and the creation of dead space will increase wound complications.
- Inadequate treatment of even minor CSF leaks may cause wound breakdown.
- Avoid inadequate stabilization; ensure there is enough structure to biomechanically fixate the spine in the face of poor bone quality and low likelihood of obtaining a true fusion.

References

Five Must-Read References

1. Patchell RA, Tibbs PA, Regine WF, et al. Direct decompressive surgical resection in the treatment of spinal cord compression caused by metastatic cancer: a randomised trial. Lancet 2005;366:643–648

2. Clarke MJ, Vrionis FD. Spinal tumor surgery management and the avoidance of complications. Cancer Control: Journal of the Moffitt Cancer Center 2014; 21(2):114–123

3. Bilsky MH, Fraser JF. Complication avoidance in vertebral column spine tumors. Neurosurg Clin N Am 2006;17:317–329, vii

4. Guzman R, Dubach-Schwizer S, Heini P, et al. Preoperative transarterial embolization of vertebral metastases. Eur Spine J 2005;14:263–268

5. Loblaw DA, Mitera G, Ford M, Laperriere NJ. A 2011 updated systematic review and clinical practice guideline for the management of malignant extradural spinal cord compression. Int J Radiat Oncol Biol Phys 2012;84:312–317

6. Quiñones-Hinojosa A, Lyon R, Ames CP, Parsa AT. Neuromonitoring during surgery for metastatic tumors to the spine: intraoperative interpretation and management strategies. Neurosurg Clin N Am 2004; 15:537–547

7. Guerin P, El Fegoun AB, Obeid I, et al. Incidental durotomy during spine surgery: incidence, management and complications. A retrospective review. Injury 2012;43:397–401

8. Chang DW, Friel MT, Youssef AA. Reconstructive strategies in soft tissue reconstruction after resection of spinal neoplasms. Spine 2007;32:1101–1106

9. Demura S, Kawahara N, Murakami H, et al. Surgical site infection in spinal metastasis: risk factors and countermeasures. Spine 2009;34:635–639

10. Wise JJ, Fischgrund JS, Herkowitz HN, Montgomery D, Kurz LT. Complication, survival rates, and risk factors of surgery for metastatic disease of the spine. Spine 1999;24:1943–1951

11. Itshayek E, Yamada J, Bilsky M, et al. Timing of surgery and radiotherapy in the management of metastatic spine disease: a systematic review. Int J Oncol 2010;36:533–544

12. Vitaz TW, Oishi M, Welch WC, Gerszten PC, Disa JJ, Bilsky MH. Rotational and transpositional flaps for the treatment of spinal wound dehiscence and infections in patient populations with degenerative and oncological disease. J Neurosurg 2004;100(1, Suppl Spine):46–51

13. Klekamp J, Samii H. Surgical results for spinal metastases. Acta Neurochir (Wien) 1998;140:957–967

14. Laufer I, Hanover A, Lis E, Yamada Y, Bilsky M. Repeat decompression surgery for recurrent spinal metastases. J Neurosurg Spine 2010;13:109–115

Index

Page numbers followed by *f* or *t* indicate figures or tables, respectively.